Award Guide
First Aid

Training guide for First Aid, CPR,
and AED Programs

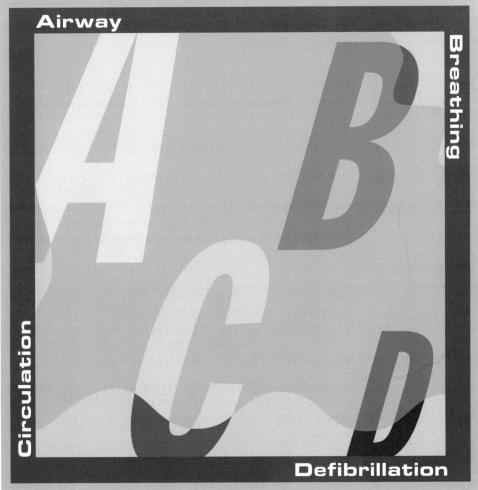

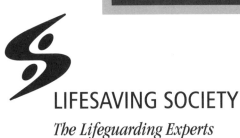

LIFESAVING SOCIETY
The Lifeguarding Experts

Canada's lifeguarding experts

– saving lives for over 100 years.

Almost 500 Canadians die every year in water-related incidents. Most of these are preventable and occur in unsupervised settings, which is why more Canadians need the basic swimming and lifesaving skills to save themselves in an aquatic emergency.

The Lifesaving Society has a long and proud history of teaching swimming and lifesaving to Canadians.

We trace our roots to the late 19th century in London, England where we began as The Swimmers' Life Saving Society. In 1894, Arthur Lewis Cochrane brought the lifesaving skills he learned in his homeland to Canada. And he passed them along to students at Upper Canada College in Toronto, Ontario. In June 1896, 18 of his students were the first recipients of our distinguished Bronze Medallion award. Under the patronage of King Edward VII in1904, we became The Royal Life Saving Society.

In the 1950s, we were the first Canadian organization to adopt mouth-to-mouth as the method of choice over manual methods of artificial respiration. We started our first CPR training program in the 1960s. In the 1980s, we initiated a project to design an economical CPR training manikin (ACTAR 911™), and we launched our Water Smart® drowning prevention campaign.

In the 1990s, the Society introduced innovative new programs including Boat Operator Accredited Training, the Junior Lifeguard Club and the Canadian Swim Patrol Program, and we launched our Aquatic Safety Management Service. We expanded our First Aid training programs and completely revamped the Bronze medal and the National Lifeguard training programs to suit the needs of the new century.

In 2001, we defined the Canadian Swim to Survive® Standard and subsequently launched our Swim to Survive program to teach Canadians the minimum essential skills they need to survive an unexpected fall into deep water. Our learn-to-swim program – Swim for Life® – is our latest drowning prevention initiative.

Today, we are known to Canadians simply as the Lifesaving Society, a national volunteer organization and registered charity. And while we've expanded our strengths over the past century to include research and public education, we haven't forgotten the ideals that formed the foundation of our organization.

The Lifesaving Society has always been – and will continue to be – Canada's lifeguarding experts.

Contents

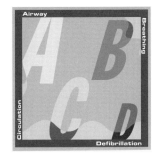

Foreword

Award Guides are designed to help instructors plan, teach, and evaluate the awards of the Lifesaving Society's training program. Award Guides should be used with the Society's *Instructor Notes,* which present essential teaching and learning principles. Instructors should consult the *Canadian First Aid Manual* or *the Canadian Lifesaving Manual* for skill descriptions and related technical information.

Each first aid certification begins with an at-a-glance overview of the general aim of the award, a list of test items, and general notes. Next, and for each test item, the Award Guide presents a detailed description including the purpose of the item, its evaluation criteria (Must Sees), and Notes:

> **Statements of Purpose**: The Purpose statements identify the objective of each item. Purpose statements define what the item achieves when performed successfully ("to restore normal breathing in a non-breathing victim") or specify why the item is included in the training program ("to demonstrate proficiency in assessing treatment priorities").

> **Notes:** The notes present explanations or limitations of the performance of an item. Suggestions to the instructor and evaluator regarding specific teaching tips or evaluation problems are also offered here. Technical information on resuscitation standards may be included. Space is often provided, for instructors to add their own additional notes. The notes include reference to the relevant content of the *Canadian Lifesaving Manual* (CLM) and the *Canadian First Aid Manual* (CFAM).

> **Performance Requirements – Must Sees**: Details of the performance which will achieve the purpose of each item are found in the Must See section. Normally, Must Sees do not describe skills or performances (skill descriptions are found in the *Canadian Lifesaving Manual* and *Canadian First Aid Manual*) and in many instances various responses are possible.

> The instructor and evaluator can use the Must Sees as a checklist for success ("victim and scene assessment", "vital signs monitored," etc.), which participants can recognize, and work on. If a candidate performs an item with the necessary knowledge, skill, and judgment to achieve its stated purpose, then he or she is probably performing at or above the required standard for the award.

The Award Guide concludes with suggested **Learning Activities.** Instructors should design or select drills, games, and other learning activities that ensure every class is action-packed, challenging, and fun.

Introduction

Helping others in need is an important social value. The desire to help and the knowledge with which to do so is a fundamental part of maintaining and regaining health in a society. Every citizen should be trained in basic life support and first aid.

First aid training provides a framework for injury prevention, emergency care, and an understanding of health. First aid training allows people to participate in their chosen endeavours with greater confidence and encourages people to contribute to their society in many valued ways.

We have learned that early access to emergency medical services to bring lifesaving assistance to an emergency can be the most important basic step. And nearly everyone can do it. It's so simple, yet makes a huge difference in the life and health of some victims.

Teaching and learning first aid

In teaching first aid, focus on the important basics – like the ABCs – that are adaptable to many varied situations, and serve as the foundation for the learning of further knowledge and skills.

Learners have their best experience when they participate fully in the acquisition of first aid knowledge, skills, and attitudes. Instructors are encouraged to use active practice-by-doing to build confidence and increase the likelihood of skill use after training.

Learners should perform the basic skills many times in training, with varied and fun practice formats. Doing once builds anxiety: doing many times builds confidence.

The 2015 resuscitation guidelines

This printing of the Lifesaving Society's *First Aid Award Guide* is updated with the most recent (2015) international resuscitation guidelines. These guidelines are designed to make it easier for first aiders and health care professionals alike to learn, remember and perform better CPR in order to maximize the chance of positive outcomes.

We have learned that continued emphasis on good and effective CPR results in better outcomes and survival rates. Good, effective CPR requires forceful, fast compressions – started as soon as possible and continued with minimal interruption. We also know that victims have a better chance when CPR is performed in combination with early defibrillation. Increasingly, first aid training will include information on the benefits of and how to use a defibrillator.

Lifesavers, lifeguards, and instructors who take and teach first aid do a great service to their family, their community, and to their country. Your first aid ability will serve you and others for a lifetime. We thank you.

Dr. Stephen B. Beerman, BSc, BSR, MD, CCFP, FCFP
Past president, International Life Saving Federation

Basic First Aid
At-a-glance

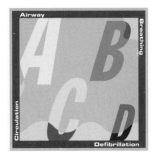

Basic First Aid covers the basics in about 3 hours including how to contact emergency medical services, rescue breathing, how to treat choking and minor injuries.

Test Items

1. Demonstrate the ability to recognize when and how to call emergency medical services (EMS).

2. Demonstrate primary assessment including hazards and ABCs of an unconscious, breathing victim.

3. Demonstrate rescue breathing with a victim of the candidate's choice or with a manikin.

4. Simulate the appearance and treatment of a conscious victim with an obstructed airway.

5. Demonstrate primary assessment and emergency care for a victim in shock.

6. Demonstrate primary assessment and appropriate care for external bleeding.

Notes

- Total estimated course time for *Basic First Aid* is about 3 hours. The actual time needed will vary with the number and maturity of the candidates, and their prior knowledge, training, and experience. Factor in additional time for refreshment and other breaks.

- Maximize practice. Limit lecture time. Candidates learn best by doing, not listening.

- In the Lifesaving Society training programs, theoretical knowledge is best measured during practical items when performance alone often reveals the extent of a candidate's knowledge. Oral evaluation techniques should be used.

- For planning and teaching Lifesaving Society First Aid Awards, refer to the detailed lesson plans and presentations featured on the Society's *First Aid Instructor Resource CD.*

- CLM reference: *Appendix B – Policy Guidelines on Rescue Breathing Practice*

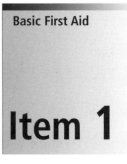

Contacting EMS

Demonstrate the ability to recognize when and how to call emergency medical services (EMS).

Purpose

To train first aiders in the appropriate procedures and reasons for contacting emergency services.

Notes

- Victim is classified as an adult. If alone, rescuer phones Emergency Medical System (EMS) right away. If another person is available, rescuer directs him or her to phone EMS.

- To help participants remember what to say when reporting an emergency, refer to the four Ws:

  Who are you? "My name is Sam Smith."

  Why are you calling? "We need an ambulance. There's been a drowning."

  What is wrong? "We found a man floating face down in the pool. He's not breathing. My friend is giving him rescue breathing."

  Where is the incident? "Send the ambulance to the backyard pool at 123 John Street. The phone number is _____."

- No coin is required to make an emergency call from a telephone booth. How to make a call may differ according to where you live. Check details in your area.

- CLM reference: *6.2 First Aid: The Rescue Process*

- CFAM reference: *p. 8 EMS*

Must See

- ❏ Basic understanding demonstrated through performance
- ❏ Candidates can give examples of circumstances requiring an EMS call
- ❏ Candidate demonstrates an EMS call providing the 4 Ws (who, why, what, where)

Primary assessment: unconscious victim

Demonstrate primary assessment including hazards and ABCs of an unconscious, breathing victim.

Purpose

To assess an unconscious breathing victim with respect to hazards and ABCs.

Notes

- Victim is classified as an adult. If alone, rescuer phones Emergency Medical System (EMS) right away. If another person is available, rescuer directs him or her to phone EMS.

- To establish unresponsiveness, rescuer may shake shoulder and ask "Are you OK?" Other techniques are acceptable.

- CLM reference: *6.4 Conduct the Primary Assessment*

- CFAM reference: p. 21-25 *Primary Assessment*

Must See

- ❏ Assessment of environment for hazards
- ❏ Establish unresponsiveness
- ❏ Activate Emergency Medical System
- ❏ Position victim (turn if necessary)
- ❏ Open airway: head-tilt/chin-lift
- ❏ Visual check for breathing (5 sec.)
- ❏ Recovery position for breathing victim

Rescue breathing

Demonstrate rescue breathing with a victim of the candidate's choice or with a manikin.

Notes

- Victim is classified as an adult. If alone, rescuer phones Emergency Medical System (EMS) right away. If another person is available, rescuer directs him or her to phone EMS.

- To establish unresponsiveness rescuer may shake shoulder and ask "Are you OK?" Other techniques are acceptable.

- Rescue breaths: rescuer delivers normal breaths (each over 1 second) that make chest rise.

- See *Canadian Lifesaving Manual*, Appendix B for guidelines on rescue breathing practice.

- CLM reference: *7.3 Coping with Complications during the ABCs*

- CFAM reference: p. 21 *ABC Priorities*; p. 25 *Special rescue breathing techniques*; p. 29 *Rescue breathing complications.*

Purpose

To restore normal breathing in a non-breathing victim.

Must See

- ❏ Assessment of environment for hazards
- ❏ Establish unresponsiveness
- ❏ Activate Emergency Medical System
- ❏ Open airway: head-tilt/chin-lift
- ❏ Visual check for breathing (5 sec.)
- ❏ 2 rescue breaths: observe chest rise
- ❏ Ability to inflate victim's lungs
- ❏ Continue rescue breathing and attempt to recuit a CPR-qualified person for assistance

Obstructed airway: conscious victim

Simulate the appearance and treatment of a conscious victim with an obstructed airway.

Purpose

To acquaint lifesavers with the appearance of a conscious victim with an obstructed airway and to introduce the appropriate lifesaving skills.

Notes

- Supervise participants carefully during training in obstructed airway techniques. Caution rescuers to *simulate* treatment: misplaced or excessive back blows or thrusts can be dangerous.

- Conscious victim simulates *either* mild *or* complete airway obstruction. To signal type of assistance needed, teach the universal choking signal.

- Rescuer assumes severe obstruction if victim nods "yes" when asked "Are you choking?" or if victim clutches neck or cannot speak or breath.

- Rescuer should assess environment for hazards.

- CLM reference: *7.3 Coping with Complications during the ABCs*

- CFAM reference: p. 30-31 *Obstructed airways - choking*

Must See

❏ Assessment of degree of obstruction – ask: "Are you choking?"
❏ Selection of appropriate procedures:

Mild obstruction

❏ Coughing encouraged
❏ Reassurance for victim

Severe obstruction

❏ Shout for help
❏ Careful landmarking
❏ Alternating back blows/abdominal thrusts until airway is clear (chest thrusts replace abdominal thrusts for pregnant or obese victim)
❏ If successful, victim directed to see physician to rule out complications from the obstruction or treatment

Shock

Demonstrate primary assessment and emergency care for a victim in shock.

Purpose

To treat and prevent further shock.

Notes

- First aiders should understand the basic causes and dangers of shock.

- The acronym W.A.R.T.S. may be a useful way to remember the key treatment priorities:
  W – Warmth
  A – ABCs
  R – Rest & reassurance
  T – Treatment
  S – Semi-prone

- CLM reference: *8.2 Shock*

- CFAM reference: p. 35-36 *Shock*

Must See

- ❑ Assessment of environment for hazards
- ❑ Establish responsiveness
- ❑ Assess ABCs
- ❑ Activate EMS
- ❑ Maintenance of natural warmth
- ❑ Rest and reassurance
- ❑ Semi-prone position (unless injury dictates otherwise)
- ❑ Recruit bystanders to assist rescuer

Bleeding

Item 6

Demonstrate primary assessment and appropriate care for external bleeding.

Purpose

To prevent further blood loss.

Notes

- First aiders should understand some causes and dangers of external bleeding.

- Design situations based on simple, real-world injuries that lifesavers are likely to encounter such as nosebleeds, scrapes and cuts. (Injury will *not* include embedded object.)

- First aiders should develop and practice simple strategies to avoid or minimize direct contact with victim's blood (e.g., improvise using T-shirt, towel or other cloth).

- CLM reference: *8.5 Bleeding*

- CFAM reference: p. 48-49 *Wounds;* p. 50 *Bandaging;* p. 62 *Nosebleeds and nose injuries*

Must See

- ❏ Assessment of environment for hazards
- ❏ Establish responsiveness
- ❏ Assess ABCs
- ❏ Check for obvious signs of bleeding
- ❏ Direct pressure
- ❏ Rest and reassurance for victim
- ❏ Recruit bystanders to assist rescuer
- ❏ Activate EMS (if required)

Emergency First Aid
At-a-glance

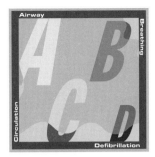

Emergency First Aid provides a general knowledge of first aid principles and the emergency treatment of injuries including: victim assessment, CPR, choking, and what to do for external bleeding, heart attack, stroke, wounds and burns. Includes CPR-B certification.

Notes

- The minimum course time required for *Emergency First Aid* is 8 hours, based on a class of 12 - 16 candidates. The actual time needed will vary with the number and maturity of the candidates, and their prior knowledge, training, and experience. Factor in additional time for refreshment and other breaks.

- See Emergency First Aid test, p. 81

- For planning and teaching Lifesaving Society First Aid Awards, refer to the detailed lesson plans and presentations featured on the Society's *First Aid Instructor Resource CD*.

- CLM reference: *Appendix B – Policy Guidelines on Rescue Breathing Practice*

Test Items

1. Through practical activities wherever possible, demonstrate an understanding of the goals of first aid.

2. Through practical activities wherever possible, demonstrate an understanding of the legal implications of providing first aid treatment.

3. Through practical activities wherever possible, demonstrate an understanding of the principles of universal precautions, including barrier devices, washing hands, and use of gloves.

4. Through practical activities wherever possible, demonstrate an understanding of the anatomy and physiology of the ABC priorities.

5. Demonstrate primary assessment of a victim including:
   - scene survey
   - level of consciousness
   - airway, breathing, circulation
   - major bleeding
   - mechanism of injury

   Demonstrate secondary assessment of a victim including:
   - vital signs
   - head-to-toe examination
   - history

6. Demonstrate one-rescuer adult, child and infant cardiopulmonary resuscitation on a manikin and how to use an AED.

7. Simulate the treatment of:
   - a conscious adult, child and infant with an obstructed airway
   - complications: a pregnant woman and person who is obese

8. Simulate the treatment of an unconscious adult, child and infant with an obstructed airway.

9. Demonstrate the effective direction of bystanders to activate EMS.

10. Demonstrate the recognition and care of a victim suffering from the following respiratory emergencies:
    - hyperventilation
    - asthma

11. Demonstrate the recognition and care of a victim suffering from:
    a) shock
    b) heart attack or angina
    c) external bleeding
    d) stroke / transient ischemic attack

12. Demonstrate the recognition and care of a victim suffering:
    a) abdominal injury
    b) burn injury
    c) facial injury

13. Demonstrate the recognition and care of an unconscious victim. Victim types should include fainting.

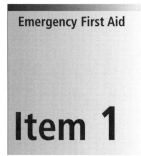

Goals of first aid

Through practical activities wherever possible, demonstrate an understanding of the goals of first aid.

Purpose

To apply first aid goals in the assessment and treatment of victims.

Notes

- Use the 3 Ps to remember the goals of first aid:
  - Preserve life
  - Prevent further injury
  - Promote recovery
- Candidates should be taught to improvise when first aid equipment and supplies are not available.
- CLM reference: *6.1 Introduction in First Aid: The Rescue Process*
- CFAM reference: p. 2 *Goals of first aid*

Must See

❑ Understanding of first aid goals demonstrated through prioritization of assessment and treatment

Legal implications of first aid

Item 2

Through practical activities wherever possible, demonstrate an understanding of the legal implications of providing first aid treatment.

Purpose

To evaluate candidate's understanding of the legal implications of providing first aid treatment.

Notes

- Candidates should be familiar with "Good Samaritan" legislation in their province or territory.
- First aiders obtain permission from parent or guardian for child or infant victims.
- Unconsciousness is implied consent.
- CLM reference: *Does the victim want your help* in *4.3 Victim Recognition;* and *Making First Contact with Victims* in *6.5 Get a History of the Victim and the Emergency*
- CFAM reference: p. 4 *First aiders and the law*

Must See

- ❏ Candidate obtains permission before beginning treatment
- ❏ Candidate can describe when treatment may be stopped

Self-protection

Item 3

Through practical activities wherever possible, demonstrate an understanding of the principles of universal precautions, including barrier devices, washing hands, and use of gloves.

Purpose

To protect the rescuer from disease transmission.

Notes

- Candidates should don gloves for bleeding or fluids; masks for breathing; and wash hands after treatment finished.
- Candidates should demonstrate how to safely don and remove gloves.
- Candidates should understand how to clean or dispose of contaminated equipment in accordance with local regulations, policies, and procedures.
- CLM reference: *Personal Safety in Assessments* in *6.6 Conduct the Secondary Assessment*
- CFAM reference: p. 12 *Prevention of disease*

Must See

❑ Appropriate use of barrier devices in various first aid situations

Anatomy and physiology of ABC priorities

Item 4

Through practical activities where possible, demonstrate an understanding of the anatomy and physiology of the ABC priorities.

Purpose

To apply understanding of the anatomy and physiology of the ABC priorities in the assessment and treatment of victims.

Notes

- Candidates should be taught to improvise when first aid equipment and supplies are not available.
- CLM reference: *Anatomy and Physiology of the ABC priorities* in *7.2 The ABC Priorities*
- CFAM reference: p. 20 *Recognition of ABC priorities;* p. 37 *Respiratory and circulatory systems*

Must See

❑ Understanding of anatomy and physiology of the ABC priorities demonstrated in dealing with respiratory and circulatory complications

❑ Ability to adapt to changing situations and improvise as necessary

Assessment

Demonstrate primary assessment of a victim including:
- *scene survey*
- *major bleeding*
- *level of consciousness*
- *mechanism of injury*
- *airway, breathing, circulation*

Demonstrate secondary assessment of a victim including:
- *vital signs*
- *history*
- *head-to-toe examination*

Notes

- Victim assessment is a required item for all first aid treatment items.

- This item is designed to emphasize the principles and procedures of victim assessment. Candidates are not expected to demonstrate treatment.

- Victim may be conscious or unconscious.

- Scene survey includes mechanism of injury and assessing risk of spinal injury.

- A-A-A-ABC extends the ABC priorities to help recall the steps in primary survey:

  A – Area (scene survey)

  A – Awake (level of consciousness)

  A – Ambulance (EMS)

  A – Airway

  B – Breathing

  C – Circulation

- CLM reference: *6.1 Introduction to the First Aid Rescue Process*

- CFAM reference: p. 21 *Primary assessment;* p. 40-41 *Secondary assessment*

Purpose

To demonstrate proficiency in assessing treatment priorities.

Must See

❏ Evaluation of the rescue scene

❏ Removal of / from danger

❏ Appropriate communication with victim

Primary assessment

❏ Assessment of level of consciousness

❏ Assessment of airway, breathing, circulation (bleeding, shock)

Secondary assessment

❏ Relevant history (accident, medical, personal)

❏ Taking and recording vital signs (respirations, pulse, pupils, skin color/temperature, level of consciousness)

❏ Systematic head-to-toe examination of victim

One-rescuer CPR: adult, child & infant

Item 6

Demonstrate one-rescuer adult, child and infant cardiopulmonary resuscitation on a manikin and how to use an AED.

Notes

- Send bystander to phone EMS. If alone with an adult victim, rescuer phones EMS right away. If alone with a child or infant victim, rescuer phones EMS after about 5 cycles of 30:2 compressions to breaths.

- Rescuers should understand the importance of early defibrillation and how to use an AED.

- While an AED could be used on an infant, it is not a requirement of this item. The need for defibrillation on infants is rare, and if defibrillation is needed, a manual defibrillator is preferred.

- Compressions: push hard and fast allowing chest to recoil completely between compressions.

- Use of barrier device is recommended.

- CLM reference: *7.5 Cardiopulmanary Resuscitation*

- CFAM reference: p. 27-28 *Cardiopulmanary Resuscitation (CPR)*

Purpose

To support breathing and circulation in an unconscious, non-breathing and pulseless victim.

Must See

- ❏ Assessment of environment for hazards
- ❏ Establish unresponsiveness
- ❏ Activate Emergency Medical System
- ❏ Attempt to obtain AED and recruit AED-trained responder if available
- ❏ Open airway: head-tilt/chin-lift
- ❏ Visual check for breathing (5 sec.)
- ❏ If breathing is absent or abnormal, CPR started with 30 chest compressions (or with 2 rescue breaths for drowning victims)
- ❏ CPR continued until EMS takes over treatment, or an AED-trained responder begins treatment with an AED, or the victim begins to move
- ❏ If victim begins to move, reassess ABCs and treat appropriately

AED protocol (adult/child)

- ❏ AED applied: clothing removed (chest bare), skin prepared, appropriate positioning of electrodes, and connection to defibrillator
- ❏ Appropriate response to voice prompts and machine indicators
- ❏ Victim cleared for analysis ensuring no motion or contact with others; visual check and "all clear" stated for analysis and shock
- ❏ AED prompts followed (sequence of analyze/shock, followed immediately by about 2 minutes of CPR) until EMS takes over treatment, or victim begins to move

Obstructed airway: conscious victim

Simulate the treatment of:
- *a conscious adult, child and infant with an obstructed airway*
- *complications: a pregnant woman and person who is obese*

Purpose

To acquaint lifesavers with the appearance of the conscious victim with an obstructed airway and introduce the techniques of the appropriate lifesaving skills.

Notes

- Supervise candidates carefully during training in obstructed airway techniques. Caution rescuers to *simulate* abdominal or chest thrusts: misplaced or excessive back blows or thrusts can be dangerous.

- Use a manikin, not a partner for safe teaching and practice of back blows and chest thrusts.

- Conscious victim simulates *either* mild *or* severe airway obstruction. To signal the type of assistance needed: teach the universal choking signal.

- Rescuer assumes severe obstruction if victim nods "yes" when asked " Are you choking?" or if the victim clutches neck or cannot speak or breath. For a child or infant victim, "Can I help?" is directed to a parent or caregiver if present.

- CLM reference: *7.3 Coping with Complications during the ABCs*

- CFAM reference: p. 30 *Obstructed airways - Choking*

Must See

Adult or child

❑ Assessment of degree of obstruction – ask "Are you choking?"

❑ Rescuer identifies self – "Can I help?"

❑ Selection of appropriate procedures:

Mild obstruction

❑ Coughing encouraged

❑ Reassurance for victim

Severe obstruction

❑ Shout for help

❑ Careful landmarking

❑ Alternating back blows/abdominal thrusts until airway is clear (chest thrusts replace abdominal thrusts for pregnant or obese victim)

❑ If successful, direct victim to see a physician to rule out complications from the obstruction or the abdominal thrusts

Infant

❑ Assessment of degree of obstruction

❑ Rescuer identifies self – "Can I help?"

❑ 5 back blows annd 5 chest thrusts

❑ Back blows and thrusts repeated until effective or the infant becomes unconscious

❑ If successful, caregiver directed to take victim to see a physician to rule out complications from the obstruction or the treatment

Obstructed airway: unconscious victim

Simulate the treatment of an unconscious adult, child and infant with an obstructed airway.

Purpose

To clear airway obstruction and restore normal breathing in an unconscious victim.

Notes

- Send bystander to phone EMS. If alone with an adult victim, rescuer phones EMS right away. If alone with a child or infant victim, rescuer phones EMS after about 5 cycles of 30:2 compressions to breaths.

- If an Automated External Defibrillator (AED) and AED-trained responder are available, rescuer should send for them after activating EMS and assist the AED responder as directed.

- If practicing this skill item on a person (versus a manikin) rescuers *simulate* compressions to prevent injury.

- Victim simulates severe airway obstruction.

- Candidates should also practice a sequence that begins with a conscious victim who becomes unconscious.

- Use of barrier device is recommended.

- CLM reference: *7.3 Coping with Complications during the ABCs.*

- CFAM reference: p. 31 *Airway obstruction procedures - conscious and unconscious*

Must See

- ❏ Assessment of environment for hazards
- ❏ Establish unresponsiveness
- ❏ Activate Emergency Medical System
- ❏ Attempt to obtain AED and recruit AED-trained responder if available
- ❏ Open airway: head-tilt/chin lift
- ❏ Visual check for breathing (5 sec.)
- ❏ If breathing is absent or abnormal, 30 chest compressions
- ❏ Attempt to ventilate

If successful:

- ❏ Continue CPR sequence

If unsuccessful:

- ❏ Reposition airway and re-attempt to ventilate
- ❏ Careful landmarking and 30 chest compressions
- ❏ Foreign body check: look in mouth and if object can be seen, attempt to remove it.
- ❏ Attempt to ventilate. Repeat sequence (reposition head, re-attempt to ventilate, chest compressions, foreign body check) until successful

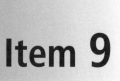

Management of bystanders

Item 9

Demonstrate the effective direction of bystanders to activate EMS.

Purpose

To direct bystanders effectively.

Must See

❏ Identification of specific bystander(s)

❏ Effective two-way communication with bystander

❏ Give clear direction: call EMS, location, number of victims, victim condition, reporting back

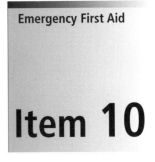

Respiratory emergencies

Item 10

Demonstrate the recognition and care of a victim suffering from the following respiratory emergencies:
- *hyperventilation*
- *asthma*

Purpose

To provide care and treatment to support breathing and encourage the return of normal breathing patterns.

Notes

Asthma:

- Candidate should determine history.

- Candidate demonstrates an understanding of the recognition and assessment of asthmatic condition.

- Candidate demonstrates an awareness of "relaxed breathing" as a form of treatment (e.g. using diaphragm inhale through nose, hold, exhale through mouth and repeat).

- Activate EMS if victim deteriorates or becomes unconscious.

- CLM reference: *8.3 Airway and Breathing Problems*

- CFAM reference: p. 33 *Asthma*; p. 33 *Hyperventilation*

Must See

❑ Determination of cause (and removal if possible) of emergency

❑ Victim and scene assessment

❑ EMS activated if necessary

❑ Individual placed in most comfortable position

❑ Victim reassured

❑ Airway and respiration maintained

Asthma

❑ Victim assisted with medication (inhaler)

Hyperventilation

❑ Encouragement of pursed lip breathing

Circulatory emergencies: shock

Demonstrate the recognition and care of a victim suffering from shock.

Purpose

To provide care and treatment to support breathing and circulation.

Notes

- Recovery position maintains an open airway and stable head position.
- Victims can be kept warm with blankets or direct body contact.
- Vital signs monitored include ABCs, skin colour and temperature, and pupils.
- CLM reference: *8.4 Circulatory Disorders*
- CFAM reference: p. 35 *Shock*

Must See

- ❏ Victim and scene assessment
- ❏ EMS activated
- ❏ Victim reassured
- ❏ Victim placed in position of comfort, preferably recovery position
- ❏ Victim kept warm
- ❏ Vital signs monitored

Circulatory emergencies: heart attack or angina

Item 11b

Demonstrate the recognition and care of a victim suffering from heart attack or angina.

Purpose

To provide care and treatment to support breathing and circulation.

Notes

- Signs and symptoms for a heart attack may include:

  - pain in chest, back, arm, neck, shoulder and/or jaw

  - nausea, vomiting and/or indigestion

  - shortness of breath, pallor, sweating, fatigue

  - apprehension, fear, denial

  Any combination of these signs and symptoms makes the possibility of heart attack more likely.

- CLM reference: *8.4 Circulatory Disorders*

- CFAM reference: p. 34 *Angina and heart attack;* p. 44 *Helping with medication*

Must See

- ❏ Victim and scene assessment
- ❏ EMS activated
- ❏ Rescuer has victim stop activity and sit or lay in a position most comfortable for the victim
- ❏ Victim reassured
- ❏ Vital signs monitored
- ❏ Medical history requested (e.g. cardiovascular disease)
- ❏ Victim helped to take medication (e.g. nitroglycerine) if available; rescuer does not administer

Circulatory emergencies: external bleeding

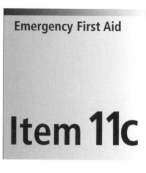

Demonstrate the recognition and care of a victim suffering from external bleeding.

Purpose

To provide care and treatment to support breathing and circulation.

Notes

- Use of tourniquets is not required for this item. However, candidates should understand the purpose of a tourniquet (e.g., apply when direct pressure fails to stop life-threatening external limb bleeding).

- Candidates should be prepared to provide own dressing and bandage; sterile dressing may be simulated.

- May include embedded objects.

- If available, rescuers should use barrier devices such as gloves and glasses to avoid exposure to blood and other body fluids.

- CLM reference: *8.5 Bleeding*

- CFAM reference: p. 48 *Wounds;* p. 50 *Bandaging;* p. 62 *Nosebleeds and nose injuries*

Must See

- ❏ Victim and scene assessment
- ❏ EMS activated if necessary
- ❏ Application of dressing and bandage
- ❏ No aggravation of injury
- ❏ Distal circulation check
- ❏ Direct pressure over wound or around wound if contains impaled object
- ❏ Reassurance for victim and instruction to rest

Circulatory emergencies: stroke/TIA

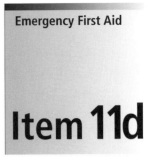

Demonstrate the recognition and care of a victim suffering from stroke / transient ischemic attack (TIA).

Purpose

To provide care and treatment to support breathing and circulation.

Notes

- Basic understanding of causes of stroke:
  - head injury
  - blood vessel blockage or burst
  - air embolism caused by injection or scuba diving
- Candidate should understand the variety of signs and symptoms that might be expressed (e.g. inability to speak, facial paralysis; limb paralysis, sensory sensations, dizziness).
- TIA - temporary stroke symptoms under 20 minutes duration. Victim should be encouraged to seek medical attention: many TIA victims may eventually suffer a stroke.
- CLM reference: *8.4 Circulatory Disorders*
- CFAM reference: p. 35 *Stroke*

Must See

- ❑ Victim and scene assessment
- ❑ EMS activated
- ❑ Victim placed in recovery position or position of comfort
- ❑ Vital signs monitored
- ❑ Victim reassured

Abdominal injury

Demonstrate the recognition and care of an abdominal injury.

Purpose

To demonstrate appropriate care of an abdominal injury.

Notes

- Assessment should consider mechanism of injury and risk of spinal injury.
- Injuries may include:
  - wounds to abdominal wall
  - blunt abdominal injury (organs protruding or not protruding)
- CLM reference: *8.5 Chest Wounds; Internal Abdominal Bleeding in 8.5 Bleeding*
- CFAM reference: p. 62-63 *Chest and abdominal injuries*

Must See

- ❏ Victim and scene assessment
- ❏ EMS activated
- ❏ Victim reassured
- ❏ Victim placed in a comfortable position with as little movement as possible until help arrives
- ❏ External bleeding (if present) controlled and wounds dressed

Burn injury

Demonstrate the recognition and care of a burn injury.

Purpose

To demonstrate the appropriate care of a burn injury.

Notes

- Cool water (10 - 25 degrees C) is best for flushing and cooling burns. Ice and ice water are not recommended.

- All electrical shock victims should be sent for medical assessment.

- CLM reference: *8.7 Burns*

- CFAM reference: p. 67-70 *Burns*

Must See

- ❏ Victim and scene assessment
- ❏ EMS activated if necessary
- ❏ Victim removed from source of injury
- ❏ Burn site immediately cooled with cool water
- ❏ Injury covered with clean (preferably sterile) dressings

Wet chemical burns
- ❏ Flushed with lots of water

Dry chemical burns
- ❏ Dust before flushing with water

Electrical burns
- ❏ Check for entry and exit burns, immobilize affected limbs

Facial injury

Demonstrate the recognition and care of a facial injury.

Purpose

To demonstrate appropriate care of a facial injury.

Notes

- Injuries may include:
  - foreign body in the ear or nose
  - laceration or contusion of eyes
  - chemical splashes in eyes
  - puncture or abrasion of eyes
  - burns to eyes
  - bleeding and fluid from ear
  - broken tooth
  - loose and displacement of tooth - laceration to mouth
  - nose bleed
  - broken nose
- CLM reference: *Nosebleed* in *8.4 Circulatory Disorders; Eye Injuries* in *8.6 Trauma Injuries*
- CFAM reference: p. 61-62 *Facial injuries*

Must See

- ❏ Victim and scene assessment
- ❏ EMS activated if necessary
- ❏ Determination of (and, if possible, removal from) cause of injury
- ❏ Selected treatment appropriate for the injury

Care of unconscious victim

Demonstrate the recognition and care of an unconscious victim. Victim types should include fainting.

Purpose

To protect the airway and provide care for an unconscious victim.

Notes

- This is a good opportunity to practice primary and secondary assessments and recovery positions.
- Fainting victims should be directed to seek medical follow-up.
- Stress the importance of good victim simulation: eyes closed, complete limpness, no movement.
- CFAM reference: p. 40-41 *Secondary Assessment;* p. 47 *Fainting*

Must See

- ❏ Victim and scene assessment
- ❏ EMS activated if necessary
- ❏ Victim placed in recovery position (except if suspected spinal injury or if moving victim will aggravate injuries)
- ❏ Airway maintained
- ❏ Rescuer looks for reason for unconsciousness (e.g. Medic Alert tag, syringe, environmental factors such as heat)

Standard First Aid
At-a-glance

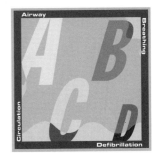

Standard First Aid provides comprehensive training covering all aspects of first aid. Standard First Aid incorporates Emergency First Aid and is designed for those who require a more in-depth understanding of first aid including: legal implications of first aid treatment, spinal injuries, heat or cold injuries, bone and joint injuries, chest injuries, and medical emergencies. Includes CPR-C certification.

Notes

- The minimum course time required for *Standard First Aid* is 16 hours, based on a class of 12 - 16 candidates. The actual time needed will vary with the number and maturity of the candidates, and their prior knowledge, training, and experience. Factor in additional time for refreshment and other breaks.

- For planning and teaching Lifesaving Society First Aid Awards, refer to the detailed lesson plans and presentations featured on the Society's *First Aid Instructor Resource CD.*

- CLM reference: *Appendix B – Policy Guidelines on Rescue Breathing Practice*

Test Items

Standard First Aid includes the Emergency First Aid Items (p. 9 – 27) in addition to the following:

1. Demonstrate two-rescuer adult, child and infant cardiopulmonary resuscitation on a manikin.

2. Demonstrate the recognition and care of a victim with a suspected spinal injury on land.

3. Demonstrate the recognition and care of a victim suffering from:
   - heat cramps, heat exhaustion, and heat stroke
   - hypothermia and frostbite

4. Demonstrate the recognition and care of a bone or joint injury.

5. Demonstrate the recognition and care of a chest injury.

6. Demonstrate the recognition and care of a head injury.

7. Demonstrate the recognition and care of a seizure victim.

8. Demonstrate the recognition and care of a diabetic emergency.

9. Demonstrate the recognition and care of a victim suffering from suspected poisoning.

10. Demonstrate an understanding of the effects of stress on victims, rescuers, and bystanders, as well as the consequences of an unsuccessful rescue.

Two-rescuer CPR: adult, child & infant

Demonstrate two-rescuer adult, child and infant cardiopulmonary resuscitation on a manikin.

Notes

- Two-rescuer CPR: both rescuers are trained. Two options: rescuers take turns doing one-rescuer CPR, or one rescuer performs chest compressions while the other does rescue breathing. Rescuers switch roles approximately every 2 minutes (5 cycles of 30:2) to minimize fatigue. Rescuers communicate and cooperate in decision-making and CPR/AED performance.

- CFAM reference: *7.5 Cardiopulmonary Resuscitation*

- CFAM reference: p. 23 *Two rescuer CPR*

Purpose

To support breathing and circulation in an unconscious, non-breathing, and pulseless victim.

Must See

Rescuer # 1

❏ Assessment of environment for hazards

❏ One-rescuer CPR sequence

Rescuer # 2

❏ Identifies self as CPR trained & confirms EMS activation

Both rescuers

❏ Continue CPR and switch roles with as little interruption as possible

❏ CPR continued until EMS takes over, or an AED-trained responder begins treatment with an AED unit, or the victim begins to move

❏ If the victim begins to move, ABCs reassessed and appropriate treatment

AED protocol (adult/child)

❏ Communication and coordination between rescuers throughout the AED protocol

❏ AED applied: clothing removed (chest bare), skin prepared, appropriate positioning of electrodes, and connection to defibrillator

❏ Appropriate response to voice prompts and machine indicators

❏ Victim cleared for analysis ensuring no motion or contact with others; visual check and "all clear" stated for analysis and shock

❏ AED prompts followed (sequence of analyze/shock, followed immediately by about 2 minutes of CPR) until EMS takes over treatment, or victim begins to move

Suspected spinal injury

Demonstrate the recognition and care of a victim with a suspected spinal injury on land.

Purpose

To provide emergency care for a victim with a suspected spinal injury on land.

Notes

- Victim may be breathing or non-breathing at the evaluator's discretion.

- Recognition is based on mechanism of injury revealed in environmental clues and/or bystander testimonials.

- For this item, candidates are not required to place the victim on a spineboard.

- CLM reference: *5.10 Rescue Procedures for Spinal Injuries*

- CFAM reference: p. 53 *Spinal injuries*

Must See

- ❏ Quick, accurate recognition
- ❏ Victim and scene assessment
- ❏ EMS activated
- ❏ Victim immobilization
- ❏ Conscious victim reassured and directed not to move
- ❏ Movement of victim minimized throughout – if movement required, immobilize spine during movement
- ❏ Appropriate care of victim throughout

Environmental emergencies: heat or cold illness

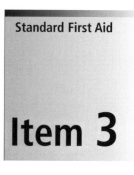

Demonstrate the recognition and care of a victim suffering from:
- *heat cramps, heat exhaustion, and heat stroke*
- *hypothermia and frostbite*

Purpose

To provide care and treatment, including the prevention of deterioration of victim condition for a victim suffering from an environmental emergency; To attempt to restore normal body temperature.

Notes

- Victims with impaired consciousness or who are unresponsive are in an immediately life-threatening condition and require immediate EMS activation.
- CLM reference: *8.9 Heat/Cold Disorders*
- CFAM reference: p. 74-76 *Action: Environmental illness and injury*

Must See

- ❏ Victim and scene assessment
- ❏ Victim reassured
- ❏ Determination of cause of injury and removal from cause
- ❏ EMS activated if necessary

Heat illness

- ❏ Victim cooled and attempt to reduce core temperature

Cold illness

- ❏ Attempt to increase core temperature

Frostbite

- ❏ Protection from further injury – apply dressing and keep warm

Bone or joint injury

Item 4

Demonstrate the recognition and care of a bone or joint injury.

Purpose

To demonstrate appropriate care of a bone or joint injury.

Notes

- Prepare candidates to recognize open and closed fractures, sprains and/or dislocations; and explore situations or mechanisms that may have caused the injury.

- Body part injured may include: clavicle, shoulder, elbow, upper or lower arm, wrist/hand, fingers, pelvis, upper or lower leg, knee, lower leg, ankle/foot, toes.

- CLM reference: *8.10 Bone, Joint, and Soft-Tissue Disorders*

- CFAM reference: p. 64-66 *Bone and joint injuries*

Must See

- ❑ Victim and scene assessment
- ❑ EMS activated if necessary
- ❑ Immobilization of injury site
- ❑ Check for sensation and circulation above and below the injury
- ❑ Treatment of wounds associated with the injury
- ❑ If available, ice applied to injury site

Chest injury

Demonstrate the recognition and care of a chest injury.

Purpose

To demonstrate appropriate care of a chest injury.

Must See

- ❏ Victim and scene assessment
- ❏ EMS activated
- ❏ Victim reassured
- ❏ Victim placed in a comfortable position with as little movement as possible until help arrives
- ❏ External bleeding (if present) controlled and wounds dressed

Suspected head injury

Demonstrate the recognition and care of a head injury.

Purpose

To demonstrate appropriate care of a head injury.

Must See

- ❏ Victim and scene assessment
- ❏ EMS activated if necessary
- ❏ Spinal immobilization if appropriate – consider risk of spinal injury
- ❏ Bandaging if situation requires (i.e. if no bleeding/discharge, no bandage required)
- ❏ Vital signs monitored
- ❏ Treatment with injured side down

Seizure

Demonstrate the recognition and care of a seizure victim.

Purpose

To demonstrate appropriate care of a seizure victim.

Notes

- Candidate should be aware of different types of seizures and appearance of each (e.g. tonic - clonic; absence).

- First aiders will usually recognize convulsive type seizures like tonic-clonic. Recognition of non-convulsive seizures like absence may be more difficult.

- Candidate should be aware of the circumstances that may cause a seizure (e.g. lack of sleep, medication, light, drugs or alcohol abuse, high temperature, head injury, diabetes).

- Candidate should recognize there may be other injuries as a result of seizure (e.g. hitting objects).

- CLM reference: *Tonic-Clonic Seizures* in *8.8 Medical Disorders*

- CFAM reference: p. 46 *Seizures;* p. 47 *Fevers in infants and children*

Must See

- ❏ Victim and scene assessment
- ❏ EMS contacted if necessary
- ❏ Recognition of seizure
- ❏ Protection of head
- ❏ Rescuer does not restrain or immobilize victim or put anything into the victim's mouth
- ❏ Removal of dangers to victim
- ❏ Victim placed in recovery position after seizure has stopped

Diabetes

Demonstrate the recognition and care of a diabetic emergency.

Purpose

To demonstrate appropriate care of a diabetic emergency.

Notes

- Candidates need not be able to distinguish between hypo-glycemia and hyperglycemia.

- Candidates should be aware that the victim may have a test kit and conscious victims should be encouraged to use the kit and take glucose if blood sugar is low.

- CLM reference: *8.8 Medical Disorders*

- CFAM reference: p. 46 *Diabetes*

Must See

- ❏ Victim and scene assessment
- ❏ EMS activated if victim is unconscious or if conscious victim does not improve
- ❏ Recognition of situation through symptoms and medical history
- ❏ Sugar administered if victim is conscious

Poisoning

Demonstrate the recognition and care of a victim suffering from suspected poisoning.

Purpose

To demonstrate appropriate care of a victim suffering from suspected poisoning.

Notes

- Candidate should be aware of the various ways a poison may enter the body:
  - injected (drug abuse, insect sting)
  - absorbed (lead)
  - inhaled (gases, drug abuse)
  - ingested (food, drug abuse)
- Some victims may suffer from an allergic reaction and may carry an auto-injector (e.g., an EpiPen®) to treat symptoms of anaphylaxis.
- With reference to the *First Aid Instructor Resource CD* (Standard First Aid Lesson Plans; Poisons) demonstrate the recognition of anaphylaxis and first aid treatment including the appropriate use of an auto-injector.
- CLM reference: *8.3 Airway and Breathing Problems*
- CFAM reference: p. 71 *Poisoning;* p. 72 *Stings & Bites;* p. 45 *Severe allergies (anaphylaxis)*

Must See

- ❏ Victim and scene assessment
- ❏ EMS activated if necessary
- ❏ Determination of cause of poisoning: identification and collection of sample (and container) of substance if feasible
- ❏ Avoidance of exposure to the poison
- ❏ Poison Control Center or EMS contacted for treatment information
- ❏ Vital signs monitored

Critical incident stress management

Demonstrate an understanding of the effects of stress on victims, rescuers, and bystanders, as well as the consequences of an unsuccessful rescue.

Purpose

To educate candidates on the implications of critical incident stress.

Notes

- CLM reference: *Appendix A – Stress Reactions to Rescues*
- CFAM reference: p. 13 *Critical incident stress*

Must See

- ❏ Awareness that critical incident stress is a normal response to an emergency
- ❏ Knowledge of where and how to access support in candidate's community

Anaphylaxis Rescuer
At-a-glance

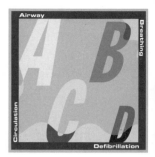

Anaphylaxis awareness has grown significantly in school boards, municipal recreation centres, camps, day care centres and among the general public. With proper training, people can learn to use an auto-injector with confidence. The recognition and first aid treatment for anaphylaxis is covered in both the Anaphylaxis Rescuer and Standard First Aid certifications; in addition the Anaphylaxis Rescuer award covers prevention and risk management. The Anaphylaxis Rescuer certification is delivered in a one-hour time frame, ideal for annual review of skills similar to CPR or combined with other first aid awards.

Notes

- The suggested course time required for the Anaphylaxis Rescuer award is 1 hour, based on a class of 12-16 candidates. The actual time needed will vary with the number and maturity of the candidates, and their prior knowledge, training, and experience. Factor in additional time for refreshment and other breaks.

- For planning and teaching Anaphylaxis Rescuer, refer to the detailed lesson plans and presentations featured on the Society's *First Aid Instructor Resource CD.*

Test Items

1. Demonstrate an understanding of:
   - what anaphylaxis is
   - recognizing an anaphylaxis victim
   - importance of early recognition and treatment
   - types of auto-injectors available and differences
   - prevention and risk management of anaphylaxis

2. Through practical activities whenever possible, demonstrate an understanding of the legal implications of providing first aid treatment.

3. Demonstrate the ability to manage an emergency scene (recognize, assess and act) and how to call emergency medical services (EMS).

4. Demonstrate the recognition and care of a victim suffering anaphylaxis reaction.

Anaphylaxis knowledge

Demonstrate an understanding of:

- *what anaphylaxis is*
- *recognizing an anaphylactic reaction*
- *importance of early recognition and treatment*
- *types of auto-injectors available and differences*
- *prevention and risk management of anaphylaxis*

Notes

- Epinephrine is a hormone produced in the body by the adrenal glands. It increases heart rate, diverts blood to the muscles, constricts blood vessels and opens the airways. Using an auto-injector is a faster means of providing epinephrine.

- It is recommened that anaphylactic or potentially anaphylactic people carry their epinephrine with them at all times since reactions can occur rapidly.

- A conservative estimate (from Food Allergy Canada) is that 2% of the population (approximately 600,000 Canadians) may be affected by potentially life-threatening allergies. The incidence may be higher in children and it has increased dramatically in the last decade.

- CFAM reference: p. 45, p. 73 *Anaphylaxis*

Purpose

To emphasize the lifesaving principles of the practical items in this award.

Must See

❏ Understanding demonstrated through performance and decision-making

Legal implications of first aid

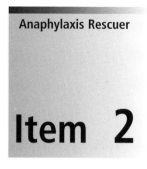

Through practical activities whenever possible, demonstrate an understanding of the legal implications of providing first aid treatment.

Purpose

To evaluate candidates' understanding of the legal implications of providing first aid treatment.

Must See

❑ Permission obtained before begining treatment
❑ Candidate describes when treatment may be stopped

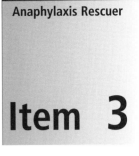

Scene management & EMS contact

Item 3

Demonstrate the ability to manage an emergency scene (recognize, assess and act) and how to call emergency medical services (EMS).

Purpose

To train first aiders in the appropriate procedures in recognizing, assessing and acting in an emergency anaphylaxis first aid situation.

Notes

- Send bystanders to phone EMS. If alone, rescuer assists the victim with auto-injector and then phones EMS right away.

- No coin is required to make an emergency call from telephone booth. How to make a call may differ according to where you live. Check for details in your area.

- CFAM reference: p. 5 *First aiders and rescue process*

Must See

❏ Basic understanding demonstrated through performance (recognize, assess, act)

❏ Candidate gives examples of circumstances requiring an EMS call

❏ A simulated call to EMS providing the 4 W's (who, why, what, where) for an anaphylactic emergency

Anaphylaxis victim

Notes

- Victim is classified as conscious adult or child victim (use only auto-injector trainers for test item). Send bystanders to phone EMS. If alone, rescuer assists victim with auto-injector and then phones EMS right away.

- Auto-injector disposal: preferably placed back into original container if available, and given to EMS upon arrival.

- Injections should be administered to the mid outer thigh. Place the tip of the auto-injector on the outer thigh and press firmly. Hold for about 10 seconds and remove. Massage injection site.

- There should be at least two doses of epinephrine available at all times. A second dose could be required 5 minutes after the first if the reaction is continuing. This situation could occur if the reaction is very severe, if the dose given is inadequate, or if the injector is faulty.

- If the victim cannot adminster his or her own auto-injector, rescuers may have to do so.

- Assist with medication: for witnessed anaphylaxis, first aiders may administer an auto-injector to an unconscious victim. E.g., the victim lost consciousness before auto-injector use. Assess level of consciousness, ABCs and initiate CPR if required.

- CFAM reference: p. 45, p. 73 *Anaphylaxis*

Demonstrate the recognition and care of a victim suffering anaphylaxis reaction.

Purpose

To respond to an anaphylactic emergency using an auto-injector.

Must See

- ❏ Recognition of victim suffering from anaphylaxis
- ❏ Assessment of enviroment for hazards
- ❏ Activate Emergency Medical System
- ❏ Consent obtained from victim or guardian
- ❏ Auto-injector obtained
- ❏ Preparation of auto-injector
- ❏ Appropriate use of auto-injector
- ❏ Safe disposal of auto-injector
- ❏ Victim reassured and placed in position of comfort
- ❏ Treatment continued until rescuer relieved of responsibility

CPR
At-a-glance

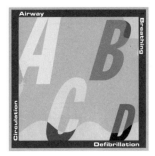

Notes

- Total estimated course time for CPR training is 3 to 8 hours. The actual time needed will vary with the level being taught (A, B or C), the number and maturity of the candidates, and their prior knowledge, training, and experience. Factor in additional time for refreshment and other breaks.

- For planning and teaching Lifesaving Society First Aid Awards, refer to the detailed lesson plans and presentations featured on the Society's *First Aid Instructor Resource CD.*

Four levels of CPR training are designed to meet the needs of both the public and professional rescuers like lifeguards:

CPR-A (Adult) teaches how to do CPR and choking procedures for adults and includes the importance of early defibrillation and how to use an AED.

CPR-B (Adult, Child & Infant) teaches parents, grandparents, babysitters, or child care workers the CPR and choking procedures for adults, children and infants. CPR-B includes the importance of early defibrillation and how to use an AED.

CPR-C (Adult, Child & Infant) covers all aspects of CPR skills and theory for adult, child and infant victims, including two-rescuer CPR skills. CPR-C includes the importance of early defibrillation and how to use an AED.

CPR-C-HCP (Adult, Child & Infant AR, AED, BVM) covers all aspects of CPR and skills and theory for adult, child and infant victims, including Rescue Breathing (artificial respiration) and the use of AEDs and BVMs. This Health Care Provider (HCP) level is designed specifically for those who as part of their job description as Health Care Providers have a duty to respond to medical emergencies (e.g. doctors, nurses, paramedics, and allied health care professionals).

Test Items

1. Demonstrate one-rescuer adult, child and infant cardiopulmonary resuscitation on a manikin and how to use an AED.

2. Demonstrate two-rescuer adult, child and infant cardiopulmonary resuscitation on a manikin.

3. Simulate the treatment of:
   - a conscious adult and child with an obstructed airway
   - complications: a pregnant woman and person who is obese

4. Demonstrate the treatment of a conscious infant with an obstructed airway on a manikin.

5. Simulate the treatment of an unconscious adult, child and infant with an obstructed airway.

6. Demonstrate rescue breathing on a manikin. (HCP only)

7. Demonstrate the use of a Bag-Valve-Mask (BVM). (HCP only)

One-rescuer CPR: adult, child & infant

Demonstrate one-rescuer adult, child and infant cardiopulmonary resuscitation on a manikin and how to use an AED.

Notes

- Send bystander to phone EMS. If alone with an adult victim, rescuer phones EMS right away. If alone with a child or infant victim, rescuer phones EMS after about 5 cycles of 30:2 compressions to breaths.

- Rescuers should understand the importance of early defibrillation and how to use an AED.

- In this item, infant AED is a requirement only for HCP candidates.

- Compression: push hard and fast allowing chest to recoil completely between compressions.

- Use of barrier device is recommended.

For HCP candidates

- Check for adequate breathing in adults and check for the presence or absence of breathing in children and infants.

- Start CPR and begin AED sequence for adults with no definite pulse, or for children with no pulse or with heart rate less than 60 bpm with signs of poor perfusion (e.g., poor colour).

- CLM reference: p. 27-28 *Cardiopulmonary resuscitation (CPR)*

- CFAM reference: p. 80-83 *AED*

Purpose

To support breathing and circulation in an unconscious, non-breathing, and pulseless victim.

Must See

- ❏ Assessment of environment for hazards
- ❏ Establish unresponsiveness
- ❏ Activate Emergency Medical System
- ❏ Attempt to obtain AED and recruit AED-trained responder if available
- ❏ Open airway: head-tilt/chin-lift

  [HCP candidates may open the airway with a jaw thrust manoeuvre if a spinal or neck injury is suspected]

- ❏ Visual check for breathing (5 sec.)
- ❏ If breathing is absent or abnormal, CPR started with 30 chest compressions (or with 2 rescue breaths for drowning victims)

  [HCP candidates check for pulse (min. 5 sec. to max. 10 sec.) before starting chest compressions]

- ❏ CPR continued until EMS takes over treatment, or an AED-trained responder begins treatment with an AED, or the victim begins to move
- ❏ If victim begins to move, reassess ABCs and treat appropriately

AED protocol (adult/child) *[HCP candidates are also evaluated on AED infant protocol]*

- ❏ AED applied: clothing removed (chest bare), skin prepared, appropriate positioning of electrodes, and connection to defibrillator
- ❏ Appropriate response to voice prompts and machine indicators
- ❏ Victim cleared for analysis ensuring no motion or contact with others; visual check and "all clear" stated for analysis and shock
- ❏ AED prompts followed (sequence of analyze/shock, followed immediately by about 2 minutes of CPR) until EMS takes over treatment, or victim begins to move

Two-rescuer CPR: adult, child & infant

Demonstrate two-rescuer adult, child and infant cardiopulmonary resuscitation on a manikin.

Notes

- Two-rescuer CPR: both rescuers are trained. Two options: rescuers take turns doing one-rescuer CPR, or one rescuer performs chest compressions while the other does rescue breathing. Rescuers switch roles approximately every 2 minutes (5 cycles of 30:2) to minimize fatigue. Rescuers communicate and cooperate in decision-making and CPR/AED performance.

For HCP candidates

- HCP rescuers use sets of 15 compressions to 2 breaths when two rescuers are present for children and infants. Two HCP rescuers use CPR thumb technique for infants.

- Check for adequate breathing in adults and check for the presence or absence of breathing in children and infants.

- Start CPR and begin AED sequence for adults with no definite pulse, or for children with no pulse or with heart rate less than 60 bpm with signs of poor perfusion (e.g., poor colour).

- CFAM reference: p. 23 *Two rescuer CPR*

Purpose

To support breathing and circulation in an unconscious, non-breathing, and pulseless victim.

Must See

Rescuer #1

❏ Assessment of environment for hazards

❏ One-rescuer CPR sequence

Rescuer #2

❏ Identifies self as CPR trained & confirms EMS activation

Both rescuers

❏ Continue CPR and switch roles with as little interruption as possible

❏ CPR continued until EMS takes over, or an AED-trained responder begins treatment with AED unit, or the victim begins to move

❏ If the victim begins to move, ABCs reassessed and appropriate treatment

AED protocol (adult/child)

❏ Communication and coordination between rescuers throughout the AED protocol

❏ AED applied: clothing removed (chest bare), skin prepared, appropriate positioning of electrodes, and connection to defibrillator

❏ Appropriate response to voice prompts and machine indicators

❏ Victim cleared for analysis ensuring no motion or contact with others; visual check and "all clear" stated for analysis and shock

❏ AED prompts followed (sequence of analyze/shock, followed immediately by about 2 minutes of CPR) until EMS takes over treatment, or victim begins to move

Obstructed airway: conscious victim

Simulate the treatment of:
- *a conscious adult and child with an obstructed airway*
- *complications: a pregnant woman and person who is obese*

Purpose

To acquaint lifesavers with the appearance of the conscious victim with an obstructed airway and introduce the techniques of the appropriate lifesaving skills.

Notes

- Supervise candidates carefully during training in obstructed airway techniques. Caution rescuers to *simulate* abdominal or chest thrusts: misplaced or excessive back blows or thrusts can be dangerous.

- Conscious victim simulates *either* mild *or* severe airway obstruction. To signal the type of assistance needed, teach the universal choking signal.

- Rescuer assumes severe obstruction if victim nods "yes" when asked "Are you choking?" or if victim clutches neck or victim cannot speak or breathe. For a child victim, "Can I help?" is directed to a parent or caregiver if present.

- CLM reference: *7.3 Coping with Complications during the ABCs*

- CFAM reference: p. 30-31 *Airway obstruction procedures - conscious and unconscious*

Must See

- ❏ Assessment of degree of obstruction – ask "Are you choking?"
- ❏ Rescuer identifies self – ask "Can I help?"
- ❏ Selection of appropriate procedures:

Mild obstruction

- ❏ Coughing encouraged
- ❏ Reassurance for victim

Severe obstruction

- ❏ Shout for help
- ❏ Careful landmarking
- ❏ Alternating back blows/abdominal thrusts until airway is clear (chest thrusts replace abdominal thrusts for pregnant or obese victim)
- ❏ If successful, direct victim to see a physician to rule out complications from the obstruction or the abdominal thrusts

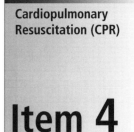

Obstructed airway: conscious infant

Item 4

Demonstrate the treatment of a conscious infant with an obstructed airway on a manikin.

Purpose

To acquaint lifesavers with the appearance of the conscious infant victim with an obstructed airway and introduce the techniques of the appropriate lifesaving skills.

Notes

- Use a manikin, not a partner, for safe teaching and practice of back blows and chest thrusts.

- For an infant victim, "Can I help?" is directed to a parent or caregiver if present.

- Assessing degree of obstruction:
  - cyanosis
  - sudden onset of breathing difficulty
  - coughing or gagging
  - high-pitched noise
  - weak cry

- With a mild airway obstruction, rescuer encourages victim's efforts to expel an obstruction naturally. If obstruction causes inadequate air exchange, rescuer performs technique for severe obstruction. Rescuer continues until successful.

- CLM reference: *7.3 Coping with Complications during the ABCs*

- CFAM reference: p. 30-31 *Airway obstruction procedures - conscious and unconscious*

Must See

- ❑ Assessment of degree of obstruction
- ❑ Rescuer identifies self – ask "Can I help?"
- ❑ 5 back blows and 5 chest thrusts
- ❑ Back blows and thrusts repeated until effective or the infant becomes unresponsive
- ❑ If successful, caregiver directed to take victim to see a physician to rule out complications from the obstruction or the treatment

Obstructed airway: unconscious victim

Simulate the treatment of an unconscious adult, child and infant with an obstructed airway.

Notes

- Send bystander to phone EMS. If alone with an adult victim, rescuer phones EMS right away. If alone with a child or infant victim, rescuer phones EMS after about 5 cycles or 30:2 compressions to breaths.
- If an Automated External Defibrillator (AED) and AED-trained responder are available, rescuer should send for them after activating EMS and assist the AED responder as directed.
- If practicing this skill item on a person (versus a manikin) rescuers *simulate* compressions to prevent injury.
- Victim simulates severe airway obstruction.
- Candidates should also practice a sequence that begins with a conscious victim who becomes unconscious.
- Use of barrier devices is recommended.

For HCP candidates

- Check for adequate breathing in adults and check for the presence or absence of breathing in children and infant.
- Start CPR and begin AED sequence for adults with no definite pulse, or for children with no pulse or with heart rate less than 60 bpm with signs of poor perfusion (e.g., poor colour).

  CLM reference: *7.3 Coping with Complications during the ABCs*
- CFAM reference: p. 30-31 *Airway obstruction procedures - conscious and unconscious*

Purpose

To clear airway obstruction and restore normal breathing in an unconscious victim.

Must See

- ❏ Assessment of environment for hazards
- ❏ Establish unresponsiveness
- ❏ Activate Emergency Medical System
- ❏ Attempt to obtain AED and recruit AED-trained responder if available
- ❏ Open airway: head-tilt/chin lift

  [HCP candidates may open the airway with a jaw thrust manoeuvre if a spinal or neck injury is suspected]
- ❏ Visual check for breathing (5 sec.)
- ❏ If breathing is absent or abnormal, 30 chest compressions

  [HCP candidates check for pulse (min. 5 sec. to max. 10 sec.) before starting chest compressions]
- ❏ Attempt to ventilate

If successful:

- ❏ Continue CPR sequence

If unsuccessful:

- ❏ Reposition airway and re-attempt to ventilate
- ❏ Careful landmarking and 30 chest compressions
- ❏ Foreign body check: look in mouth and if object can be seen, attempt to remove it.
- ❏ Attempt to ventilate. Repeat sequence (reposition head, re-attempt to ventilate, chest compressions, foreign body check) until successful

Rescue breathing

Demonstrate rescue breathing on a manikin.

Purpose

To restore normal breathing in a non-breathing adult, child or infant victim.

Notes

- Check for adequate breathing in adults and check for the presence or absence of breathing in children and infants.

- Rescue breaths: rescuer delivers normal breaths (each over 1 second) that make chest rise.

- Adults – give 1 breath every 5 to 6 seconds (10 to 12 breaths per minute). Children and infants – give breath every 3 to 5 seconds (12 to 20 breaths per minute).

- CLM reference: *7.4 Rescue Breathing*

- CLM reference: *p. 22 Action priorities*

- See *Canadian Lifesaving Manual*, Appendix B for guidelines on rescue breathing practice.

Must See

- ❏ Assessment of environment for hazards
- ❏ Establish unresponsiveness
- ❏ Activate Emergency Medical System
- ❏ Open airway: use jaw-thrust manoeuvre if a spinal or neck injury is suspected
- ❏ Visual check for breathing (5 sec.)
- ❏ 2 rescue breaths: observe chest rise
- ❏ Continue rescue breathing checking pulse about every 2 minutes
- ❏ Check for pulse (no more than 10 sec.)
- ❏ If pulseless initiate CPR

Bag-Valve-Mask (BVM)

Demonstrate use of a Bag-Valve-Mask (BVM).

Purpose

To restore normal breathing in a non-breathing adult, child or infant victim with BVM.

Notes

- CFAM reference: p. 88
  Bag-valve-mask (BVM)

Must See

1-rescuer technique

❏ Rescuer positioned directly above victim's head

❏ Mask positioned correctly

❏ Use of "C-E clamp" technique to hold mask in place while lifting the jaw to open airway

❏ Effective 1 sec. ventilations (squeezing bag) causing chest to rise

2-rescuer technique

❏ First rescuer opens airway with head tilt and jaw lift, sealing mask over victim's mouth and nose

❏ Effective 1 sec. ventilations by second rescuer (squeezing bag) causing chest to rise

Automated External Defibrillation

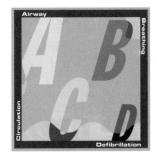

At-a-glance

Automated External Defibrillation (AED) provides knowledge of how the heart works and what goes wrong when defibrillation is required. The AED course covers: when and how to operate an AED; AED maintenance; data management and the reporting protocols required after an incident in which an AED unit is used.

Notes

- The recommended minimum course time for AED is 4-5 hours. The actual time needed varies with the number and maturity of candidates, and their prior knowledge, training, and experience. Factor in additional time for refreshment and other breaks.

- For planning and teaching Lifesaving Society First Aid Awards, refer to the detailed lesson plans and presentations featured on the Society's *First Aid Instructor Resource CD*.

AED Items

1. Demonstrate knowledge of when to use and how to operate an Automated External Defibrillator (AED), including maintenance of AED unit, data management and reporting protocols.

2. Demonstrate one- and two-rescuer adult and child automated external defibrillation on a manikin.

AED knowledge: use and operation

Demonstrate knowledge of when to use and how to operate an Automated External Defibrillator (AED), including maintenance of AED unit, data management and reporting protocols.

Purpose

To emphasize the lifesaving principles of automated external defibrillation, and develop an understanding of when and how to use an AED.

Notes

- Candidates should understand that various suppliers manufacture AED units. These units differ and require specific training prior to their use.

- Victim's chest may require drying and shaving.

- CFAM reference: p. 80-83 *Automated External Defibrillator (AED)*

Must See

❑ Understanding demonstrated through performance and decision-making

❑ Accurate and logical assessments, decisions, and conclusions

❑ Ability to activate an AED unit

❑ Ability to connect and position electrodes appropriately

❑ Ability to follow the AED prompts given

❑ Understanding of how to conduct daily maintenance and weekly time checks

❑ Understanding of the importance of conducting quarterly skill assessments

❑ Understanding of how to complete AED incident reports

One- and two-rescuer AED

Demonstrate one- and two-rescuer adult and child automated external defibrillation on a manikin.

Purpose

To respond to an emergency as a single rescuer or as a member of a team utilizing AED equipment; To restore circulation of a victim suffering from signs of pulselessness.

Must See

- ❏ Assessment of environment for hazards
- ❏ Establish unresponsiveness
- ❏ Activate Emergency Medical System
- ❏ Attempt to obtain AED and recruit AED-trained responder if available
- ❏ Open airway
- ❏ Visual check for breathing (5 sec.)
- ❏ If breathing is absent or abnormal, CPR started with 30 chest compressions (or with 2 rescue breaths for drowning victims)
- ❏ CPR started with chest compressions and continued until AED arrives
- ❏ AED applied: clothing removed (chest bare), skin prepared, appropriate positioning of electrodes on victim, and connection to defibrillator
- ❏ Appropriate response to voice prompts and machine indicators
- ❏ Victim cleared for analysis ensuring no motion or contact with others. Visual check and "all clear" stated for analysis and shock
- ❏ AED prompts followed (sequence of analyze/shock, followed immediately by about 2 minutes of CPR) until advanced health care providers take over treatment, or victim begins to move

Airway Management
At-a-glance

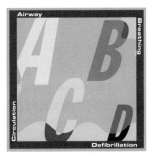

Airway Management certification provides senior and experienced lifeguards with specific knowledge and training in the use of oxygen, suction devices, oral airways and mask/bag-valve-mask (BVM).

Notes

- The minimum recommended course time for *Airway Management* is 4 to 5 hours. The actual time needed will vary with the number and maturity of the candidates, and their prior knowledge, training, and experience. Factor in additional time for refreshment and other breaks.

- For planning and teaching Lifesaving Society First Aid Awards, refer to the detailed lesson plans and presentations featured on the Society's *First Aid Instructor Resource CD.*

- CLM reference: *The Administration of Oxygen* in *8.3 Airway and Breathing Problems*

- Other reference: The Lifesaving Society's *Oxygen Administration* booklet

Test Items

1. Demonstrate an understanding of the:
   - principles of respiration and circulation
   - importance and application of universal precautions and use of barrier devices
   - purpose and use of oropharyngeal airways
   - principles and practical application of oxygen supplementation
   - purpose and use of manual suction

2. Demonstrate the proper use and application of at least one barrier device during the delivery of artificial respiration.

3. On a manikin, demonstrate the proper sizing, insertion, and follow-up for the use of an oropharyngeal airway.

4. Demonstrate understanding of the components and proper usage, including safety factors, of nasal cannula, face mask, non-breathing mask, pocket mask, and bag-valve-mask delivery systems.

5. Demonstrate the application of an oxygen delivery system to a victim in need of supplemental oxygen.

6. Demonstrate the proper use and application of a manual suction device in the treatment of a victim who is vomiting or who has fluid in the upper airway.

Knowledge

Demonstrate an understanding of the:
- *principles of respiration and circulation*
- *importance and application of universal precautions and use of barrier devices*
- *purpose and use of oropharyngeal airways*
- *principles and practical application of oxygen supplementation*
- *purpose and use of manual suction*

Purpose

To emphasize the lifesaving principles of the practical items in this award.

Notes

- Theoretical knowledge is best measured during practical items when performance alone often reveals the extent of the candidate's knowledge and understanding. A separate evaluation of knowledge may only be required for material not easily integrated into the test items.

- CFAM reference: p. 84-88 *Oxygen Administration*

Must See

❏ Understanding demonstrated through performance and decision-making

❏ Accurate and logical assessments, decisions, and conclusions

Barrier devices

Demonstrate the proper use and application of at least one barrier device during the delivery of artificial respiration.

Purpose

To emphasize the importance of universal precautions during resuscitation attempts.

Notes

- Instructors should strive to introduce candidates to as many types of barrier devices as possible including disposable and non-disposable.

- Instructors should also reinforce the importance of wearing gloves during a rescue and washing hands afterwards.

- CFAM reference: p.12 *Rescue breathing devices;* p. 85 *Mask;* p. 88 *Non-rebreathing mask*

Must See

❏ Complete universal precautions taken

❏ Appropriate use of barrier devices

❏ Ability to deal with complications such as vomiting and the return of spontaneous respiration

❏ Accurate and continuous monitoring of victim's vital signs

❏ Ability to deal with challenges such as a stoma or spinal injury

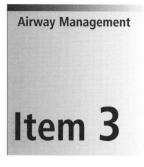

Oropharyngeal airways

On a manikin, demonstrate the proper sizing, insertion, and follow-up for the use of an oropharyngeal airway.

Purpose

To establish and maintain a patent airway in an unconscious victim.

Notes

- Instructors should demonstrate insertion techniques for both adult and infant victims.
- Every effort should be made to make manikins available for candidates.
- CFAM reference: p. 86 *Oropharyngeal airways*

Must See

- ❏ Quick, accurate recognition and reaction
- ❏ Correct and accurate sizing of airway
- ❏ Appropriate response to victim not accepting airway
- ❏ Correct insertion of airway
- ❏ Appropriate check for airway patency
- ❏ Appropriate follow-up
- ❏ Appropriate record keeping
- ❏ When appropriate, correct removal of airway
- ❏ Ability to deal with complications, i.e. vomiting, victim regaining consciousness
- ❏ Ability to deal with challenges such as a stoma or spinal injury

Oxygen delivery system

Demonstrate understanding of the components and proper usage, including safety factors, of nasal cannula, face mask, non-breathing mask, pocket mask, and bag-valve-mask delivery systems.

Purpose

To utilize various oxygen delivery systems effectively and safely.

Notes

- Stress the importance of selecting appropriately sized mask for the victim.

- CFAM reference: p. 85 *About oxygen equipment;* p. 86, 88 *Advanced Airway Management*

Must See

- ❏ Identification of different types of tanks and tank sizes
- ❏ Correct assembly of oxygen system
- ❏ Ability to read tank regulator
- ❏ Knowledge of flow rates of different delivery systems
- ❏ Demonstrated safety precautions
- ❏ Appropriate use of oxygen delivery accessories

Oxygen supplementation

Demonstrate the application of an oxygen delivery system to a victim in need of supplemental oxygen.

Purpose

To provide supplemental oxygen to a victim in respiratory distress or arrest.

Notes

- Victims are assessed with a pulse oximeter unless they have suffered a drowning incident, decompression sickness (SCUBA incident), carbon monoxide poisoning, or are in respiratory arrest.

- CFAM reference: p. 85 *About oxygen equipment;* p. 86, 88 *Advanced Airway Management*

Must See

- ❏ Appropriate choice of delivery method and flow rate for victim's condition
- ❏ Correct application of delivery method to victim
- ❏ Appropriate and continuous monitoring of victim's vital signs
- ❏ When applicable, correct removal of delivery method from victim
- ❏ Appropriate and accurate record keeping
- ❏ Appropriate follow-up
- ❏ Correct safety precautions throughout

Manual suction

Demonstrate the proper use and application of a manual suction device in the treatment of a victim who is vomiting or has fluid in the upper airway.

Purpose

To establish and maintain a patent airway in a victim whose airway is compromised by fluid.

Notes

- Instructors are encouraged to review obstructed airway procedures.
- To avoid cross-contamination, catheter tips should not be inserted into candidates' mouths.
- Candidates need to be familiar with how to deal with a blockage in the catheter.
- CFAM reference: p. 87 *Suction devicies*

Must See

- ❏ Quick, accurate recognition and reaction
- ❏ Correct and accurate sizing and insertion
- ❏ Appropriate use
- ❏ Appropriate follow-up
- ❏ Ability to deal with challenges such as a spinal injury
- ❏ Proper disposal and sanitation procedures

Learning Activities
Skill drills and
Simulated emergencies

Skill drills

Use skill drills to develop mastery of individual skills, like obstructed airway sequences for example. Ensure candidates have learned the basic skills required before asking them to apply those skills or skill sequences in a simulated emergency situation.

Simulated emergencies

Once candidates have acquired the basic first aid skills, use simulated emergency situations to develop judgment. Such emergency scenarios are an excellent way to develop candidates' problem-solving and decision-making ability.

Design the scenarios carefully to elicit the rescuer responses you wish to practice. Coach "victims" in how to most realistically simulate their condition. Use props as appropriate. Utilize bystanders, family, etc. to create realistic attitudes. Use real scenarios from newspapers, the Internet, etc.

At the outset of training, consider working through an emergency situation as a group. You might put the scenario on an overhead or flip chart, and guide the group through the problem orally.

Notes

- The experience, maturity, and proficiency of candidates may vary greatly. Adapt your course to meet the needs of your learners.

- Recruit experienced instructors to help with material with which you may need assistance. Enlist the assistance of candidates with special skills.

- Foster a positive and co-operative atmosphere for learning. Maintain a learning environment in which candidates feel comfortable about making mistakes as they learn.

- Simplify material. Focus on similarities between content areas. Integrate topics so that the overall course themes are clear.

Sample scenarios

❑ At work, you find a co-worker face down on the lunchroom floor not moving. You are alone. What do you do?

❑ You are in your backyard, when you hear your neighbour calling for help. You respond to discover your neighbour's husband lying motionless in the yard. What do you do?

❑ You are on the phone when you hear your mother screaming. You rush outside to discover she has just pulled your 2-year-old brother from the family pool. What do you do?

❑ You are driving behind a car that suddenly veers off the road and strikes a utility pole. The pole breaks, dropping wires on the now wrecked car. You stop to help. What do you do?

❑ You and your four friends are playing basketball on the driveway when two players go up for a rebound and collide. Both fall to the ground. One twists her ankle and is bleeding from the knee; the other has landed face down and is not moving. What do you do?

❑ You are walking your dog when you notice an elderly man walking towards you lose his balance and fall to the sidewalk. When you get near him, he is semi-conscious. His eyes are open and the left side of his face is drooping. The man is mumbling something but you can't understand him. Suddenly he begins to vomit. What do you do?

- *Apply* knowledge. Keep activities practical and design them so candidates must apply theoretical knowledge.

- Emphasize the basics. Teach candidates what they will *need* to know and are likely to remember in a real emergency. If knowledge doesn't affect or change what first aiders *do*, then it is probably superfluous.

- Provide lots of practice time.

- Teach first aid skills separately before combining them in simulated emergencies.

❏ After Sunday dinner, your 65-year-old aunt complains of indigestion. She says she has severe stomach pain and is sick. She blames the food for the pain and nausea. You notice that her skin is pale, her breathing rapid, and she looks ill. What do you do?

❏ Your dad is clearing leaves out of the gutters on the roof. You go into the house to answer the phone. You come out to find him face-up on the ground with the ladder lying on top of him. He is not moving and seems to be unconscious. What do you do?

❏ You are having dinner with your family at a restaurant when a man at a nearby table collapses to the floor. What do you do?

❏ You walk into your kitchen and discover your 3-year-old nephew motionless on the kitchen floor. You notice an unopened bottle of medication nearby. What do you do?

❏ You are returning to camp from a hiking trip. As you enter your campsite you notice your friend coughing and clutching her throat. You see a red swollen mark on her right arm. What do you do?

❏ You are driving your boat and notice two people in the water holding onto a capsized canoe and waving for help. What do you do?

❏ You are in a playground and see a child fall from a swing, landing face down on the ground. As the young girl gets up, you notice she is bleeding from her nose and has a cut lip. She begins to cry and screams for her mother. What do you do?

❏ You are at home when you hear a loud explosion from your backyard. As you run to see what happened, you notice your neighbour screaming in pain covering his face with both hands. A barbecue is tipped over and on fire. What do you do?

❏ You are riding the bus on a very hot and humid day. You notice an elderly man at the back wearing a suit and tie lose his balance and collapse. What do you do?

❏ You are at a party when you notice a young man collapse while dancing. His body stiffens and convulses. What do you do?

Learning Activities
Legal Implications of First Aid

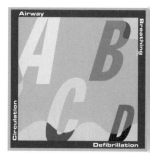

Here come da judge!

Give candidates cards outlining a role they are to play in the legal aftermath of a first aid incident. Provide adequate time to research their roles. Instructor remains neutral and guides the process.

Variations

❏ Simulate successful and non-successful rescue attempts.

❏ Utilize bystanders, family etc. to create realistic attitudes.

❏ Use real scenarios from newspapers, the Internet, etc.

Special guest

Invite a lawyer, paralegal, police officer, etc. to speak about the legal implications during a first aid incident.

Puzzler

Create a puzzle that emphasizes key aspects of legal implications in first aid. Candidates solve the puzzle individually or in groups.

Consider

❏ True/False quiz sheets, crossword puzzles, word search puzzles, candidate created puzzles.

Learning Activities
Assessment & Contacting EMS

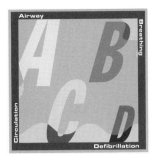

Notes

Hide & seek

Pair candidates. Half the candidates face a wall while their partners "hide" close by. Partners simulate an unconscious victim. On a signal, candidates find their partners and do a primary assessment. Ensure "hiding spots" are safe and within eyesight.

Variations

- ❏ Have candidates practice simulating unconscious victims. Are their arms and legs limp? Do they feel heavy to move or roll over? Are they unresponsive?

- ❏ Set out a telephone in the vicinity. At the end of the primary assessment, quiz pairs. Who can identify the location of the telephone? Switch roles. Repeat the activity. Change the location of the telephone.

- ❏ Include props that indicate hazards. Once again, at the end of the activity, quiz candidates to see who noticed and responded.

Step by step

Set up stations along a wall. Post a key word (or a graphic) from each Must See so that stations proceed in the order of a primary assessment. In partners, candidates take turns fulfilling the Must See requirements and then move to the next station. Include related props,

such as a telephone or items to simulate environmental hazards.

Variations

- ❏ Repeat the activity, but remove one or two of the Must See signs. Candidates move through the stations, but "fill" in the blank spaces from memory, completing the primary assessment sequence in full.

- ❏ Continue to remove Must See signs, until candidates complete the full sequence on their own.

Twenty questions

Divide candidates into 2 groups. Each group creates a rescue scenario involving a conscious and co-operative victim. They decide upon a chief complaint of the victim, and how the injury occurred. Then candidates pair up with a person from the other group. Partners try to figure out the details of each other's injury through direct questioning.

Variations

- ❏ Partners alternate questions. Each tries to be the first to figure out the details of the injury and victim type.

- ❏ Provide a telephone. When partners think they have gathered sufficient details, they simulate a call to the EMS.

(cont'd)

- Basic First Aid, Emergency First Aid, Standard First Aid, and CPR awards all include assessment of environment for hazards. Scene "freezing" after 20 to 30 sec. is a good way to emphasize this aspect.

- Teach the use of a phrase like – "No Fire, No Wire, No Gas, No Glass, Gloves & Mask, Don't forget to Ask." – as a memory cue to remind candidates to look around and assess the scene upon entering, rather than exclusively focusing on the victim.

❑ Bring partners together into a large group. Put the telephone in the centre of the circle. One candidate simulates the EMS call based on the information gathered from his or her partner. The group that designed the scenario decides whether all the details have been properly relayed. If not, then another person tries, and so on, until the call passes inspection. Then groups switch roles.

❑ Provide simple make-up kits, so groups can simulate bleeding and/or shock. Provide simple props to indicate hazards. (See 'Victim Simulation' in *Instructor Notes*.) Keep the injuries simple!

Circuit

Set up 4 stations around the teaching area. Each station features a "victim," and focuses on a different first aid item: primary assessment, rescue breathing, obstructed airway – conscious victim, and shock. Candidates travel the circuit. Supervise carefully! Emphasize safe first aid care, not speed.

Variations

❑ To ensure maximum participation from candidates, use family volunteers, helpers, or others to simulate the victims. Coach volunteers ahead of time about how to act for their role. Use simple make-up and props.

❑ Have candidates design the stations. Choose from a list of victims.

❑ After candidates have worked through the circuit once, gather them together. Give feedback about their first aid responses. Have them work through the circuit a second time aiming to improve performance.

Freeze frame

Set up a rescue scenario and provide props to indicate hazards. Thirty seconds after the rescuer has entered and initiated a rescue response, "freeze-frame" the scene. Victims and bystanders do not move, nor do conditions change. Candidates assess the situation and report their assessment of environmental hazards and the victim's condition.

Variations

❑ Repeat with new scenarios. Shorten the amount of time for assessment.

❑ Set up a situation where the victim should not be moved. Use props and positioning of the victim to indicate the type of injury.

❑ Complete the activity in two stages. First, candidates observe and assess the scene and victim. Second, candidates complete the rescue basing their response upon all of the information.

Piecing the puzzle together

Divide candidates into 2 groups, bystanders and rescuers. Give each bystander a single piece of information about the rescue scenario so that no bystander has the complete picture or the same piece of information. Include information vital to the rescue as well as information that will have no impact upon the rescue response. Rescuers quiz bystanders gathering together bits of information. They come to a conclusion about the chief complaint of the victim, and how the injury occurred.

Variations

❑ Give rescuers pencil and paper to record vital pieces of information.

❑ Follow-up by acting out the situation and/or simulating a call to the EMS to describe what has happened and the state of the victim.

- [ ] Prepare bystander cards or clues ahead of time. Bystanders draw a card containing their piece of information.

- [ ] Include picture cues as well as word descriptions. Keep information brief and simple.

- [ ] Play a modified game of Clue, focusing upon injury and how it happened rather than "whodunit."

Incident forms

Candidates perform a rescue. Stop the rescue sequence after the primary assessment stage. Then have rescuers fill out an "incident form" as completely as they are able based upon their assessment and initial actions. (See sample form in *Alert: Lifeguarding in action*, p. 80-81.) The purpose of the activity is to help candidates become aware of the types of information they need to gather, rather than evaluate ability to fill out a form.

Variations

- [ ] Gather candidates into a group. Orally work through the incident form together. Read the questions aloud and have candidates tell you the answers. Draw attention to areas where information is incomplete.

- [ ] Design a simple incident form appropriate for minor injuries and suitable to the age and skill level of the participants.

"W" cards

Make four cards. Each card features one of these words: Who, Why, What, Where. Divide candidates into groups of four and give each group a set of four cards. Groups sit in circles, with each person drawing a card. Then they simulate an emergency medical services call. The person with the "Who" card begins, stating name. The person with the "Why" card continues, stating why the call is being made. Next, the person with the "What" card adds to the

script, telling what has happened. Finally the person with the "Where" card finishes the call, stating location.

Variations

- [ ] Switch cards and roles.

- [ ] Provide telephones. Pass the receiver around the circle as a new person talks.

- [ ] Candidates make up the situations and details, showing an understanding of when to contact EMS.

Spread the word

Show candidates a newspaper article that features a successful rescue by a young person, particularly one where the youth has contacted emergency medical services. Encourage candidates to bring to class similar newspaper clippings they find. Point out actions the young rescuers took that saved lives. Where appropriate to the age and skill level, simulate the rescue in class.

Variations

- [ ] Post on a bulletin board in a prominent area.

- [ ] Include the name of the candidate who brought the newspaper clipping to class.

- [ ] Photocopy the stories, and send them home with candidates to share with their families.

I know the number

Have candidates identify the telephone number for emergency medical services (EMS) in their area. Photocopy and distribute EMS cards for candidates to place by their telephone at home or stick to their refrigerator with a magnet. Cards feature the EMS telephone number in the area and the four W's – Who, Why, What, Where.

(cont'd)

Variations

❏   Quiz candidates throughout the course of the lessons, asking them to shout aloud the EMS number.

❏   Work the task into drills and skill practice.

He went that-a-way

When setting up situations to practice emergency care or rescue breathing skills, provide candidates with actual locations in their community as part of the scenario.

Assign locations relevant to the candidates, and where accidents are more likely to occur, such as at their home, school, playground, cottage, or backyard pool.

Make contacting emergency medical services part of every emergency situation. Ensure candidates practice giving directions, and other relevant details, and do not gloss over the information by simply stating during practice "I've telephoned for help."

Wallet card

Have the candidates design a wallet or "pocket" card containing all the information they would need to know in an emergency. Provide a telephone book of the area so that candidates may look up the appropriate emergency telephone numbers.

Candidates may also make a poster of emergency telephone numbers to keep by their home telephone.

During practice, provide props such as a telephone. Evaluate candidates carefully. Check that they dial the appropriate numbers while contacting the emergency medical services. Don't be satisfied to simply see that they are making a phone call. Find out the DETAILS of that phone call!

A little help from your friends

Once candidates know how to contact the EMS themselves, have them practice sending someone else to make the call:

Variations

❏   a bystander trained in lifesaving

❏   a small child (5-6 years old)

❏   an untrained bystander

Number please?

Provide participants with a telephone book. Have them find the numbers to call in an emergency in their community. (Emergency numbers are usually listed at the front of the book).

If available, distribute stickers from local police and fire departments. Have participants fill in the blanks on the stickers with the emergency numbers.

Self-evaluation

Use a tape recorder and a blank cassette to record the "calls" so that participants can evaluate their own performance. Give participants the opportunity to improve by repeating the activity.

Script

Write a script for participants to read while contacting emergency medical services. Use a large piece of Bristol board, and post the script near the telephone. Leave blanks for the rescuer to fill in information relevant to the particular rescue. Keep the script short, and the language simple. After a while, remove the script to see if participants have absorbed the information.

Telephone know-how

Discuss the information that the emergency medical services will need to know in order to help during a rescue. Make a checklist of the information. Post it.

Divide the participants into pairs. One member of the pair is assigned the role of reporting an accident. The other member is assigned the role of receiving the call at the emergency medical services "headquarters." Have the pairs evaluate their performance using the checklist.

Switch roles.

Role play

Use the checklist as part of every rescue requiring the assistance of the emergency services. Ensure rescuers "role play" the steps, and do not simply state they are making a phone call. Provide telephones with which rescuers practice dialing the appropriate number for contacting emergency services in their community, and giving the appropriate information.

Emergency card

Provide participants with an "emergency card" to be posted by their telephone at home. Leave blanks for the participants to fill in relevant information, such as emergency telephone numbers, and address.

Learning Activities
Respiratory Emergencies

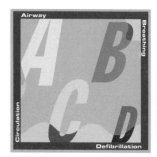

Rescue breathing

Rescue cards

Make cards with pictures that represent the steps of rescue breathing – one step per card. Laminate the cards. Scramble and spread the cards on the floor. On your signal, candidates put the cards in order.

Variations

❑ Time the activity. Repeat, challenging candidates to beat their time.

❑ Make two sets of cards. Do the activity as a team race. First team to put the cards in proper order wins!

Buddy system

Pair candidates. Each candidate takes responsibility for making sure that his or her partner can perform the sequence for rescue breathing. When pairs think they've "got it right," they demonstrate the skill for evaluation.

Variations

❑ If pairs make a mistake, review that portion of the sequence with them. Have them practice on their own again, and return for demonstration when they have practiced the sequence correctly.

❑ Encourage candidates to teach their families and friends rescue breathing.

Obstructed airway

Balloon & quarter trick

Here is a way to demonstrate the effect of applying pressure below the lungs during abdominal thrusts. Put a quarter in the neck of a balloon that has been blown up. Squeeze the balloon from bottom. The "obstruction" (quarter) pops out.

Variations

❑ Declare balloon day! Use balloons for other activities. For example, try blowing up a balloon with an obstruction in it.

Charades

Write victim types on pieces of paper and put them in a hat. Include "Mild Obstruction" and "Severe Obstruction." Candidates draw and act out a victim type. Peers shout out the type.

Variations

❑ Person who correctly shouts out the victim type is the next person to draw from the hat.

❑ Add treatment to the game. Person not only identifies victim type, but does basic treatment (simulating thrusts) according to the Must See for the item.

❑ During the "charade", call out the name of a candidate. That person shouts out the victim type and performs treatment. Repeat until everyone has had a turn identifying, treating, and simulating at least one victim type.

Notes

• Relate true-life stories where rescue breathing has saved lives.

Mini first aid competition

Set up three events based upon the award items. Include primary assessment, rescue breathing, and Obstructed Airway – Unconscious Victim. Devise a simple scoring system using the Must See requirements. Give 1 mark if requirement was attempted; 2 marks if done satisfactorily. Make fun "medals" or "trophies" for scores.

Variations

❏ Find something positive about every candidate's performance, and reward accordingly. For example, make individualized ribbons, such as "Great victim reassurance!" or "Terrific use of bystanders!"

❏ Candidates use manikins with lungs to demonstrate rescue breathing and abdominal thrusts.

Relay

Divide candidates into groups of five. One person simulates an unconscious, non-breathing victim. The others are rescuers. With the victim situated on land, at your signal the first team member runs to the victim to provide primary assessment of unconscious victim and returns to the start. The second rescuer adds rescue breathing to the sequence. The third rescuer treats for vomiting, and the fourth for obstructed airway. The victim remains unconscious throughout. Supervise carefully to ensure safe simulations.

Variations

❏ Time teams. Add 30 sec. to the result for improper treatment. Team with the lowest time wins.

❏ Give "red flags" (small strips of red cloth) to teams for each "mistake" in treatment as it is made. The winning team is not the fastest, but the one given the fewest red flags.

A star is born

The setting is Hollywood. The instructor is the casting director for a movie. The audition consists of simulating victim types. The candidate performing the most realistic simulated victim is awarded the part in the movie.

Role-playing

Divide the class into small groups. Give each group a prop. Props may include:

• empty medicine bottles

• a cord to simulate an electrical wire

• a dinner plate and fork

• a fishing rod

• a large box to simulate an old refrigerator

Challenge each group to use the prop to dramatize a cause of asphyxia and the appropriate treatment. Allow five minutes planning time.

Supervise the activity carefully. Do not allow the candidates to use the props in such a way that their own safety is endangered.

(cont'd)

Checklist

Make a master checklist on a piece of Bristol board. Show the steps in treatment of an unconscious non-breathing victim with an obstructed airway. Use the "Must Sees" to help you make the list. Post on wall.

Divide candidates into groups of three. Assign roles of victim, rescuer, and evaluator. Have the evaluator use the checklist to provide feedback to the rescuer, and shape performance, DURING the skill practice. Ensure EACH step is followed.

Emphasize that manual thrust techniques must be SIMULATED.

Memory challenge

A candidate acts out one characteristic of a conscious victim with an obstructed airway, partial blockage. The next candidate repeats that characteristic and adds another. The game continues until all the characteristics are added to the sequence. If a candidate skips a characteristic the game begins all over. Repeat the game for a conscious victim with a complete airway obstruction.

Learning Activities
Circulatory Emergencies

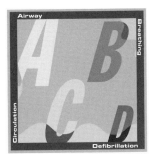

Assessing pulse & respiration rates

▋ Pulse circle!

Candidates sit in two circles, one circle inside the other. People in the outer circle locate the pulse of a person in the inner circle. Then they rotate one "space" clockwise, and repeat until they've located the pulse of each person in the inner circle.

Variations

❏ Challenge candidates to locate a pulse at the neck and the wrist. Which was easier to find?

❏ Have candidates locate and count a partner's pulse for ten seconds. What will the pulse rate be for a minute?

❏ Find pulse rates of family members as an at-home assignment.

▋ Monitor & record!

Set up a variety of tasks. Candidates measure and record their pulse for each task. Analyze the results together. Did heart rate change according to the task? How? Test pulse rates while sitting, standing, and playing a game, after a sprint, during a warm-up or cool-down, and a few minutes after a workout.

Variations

❏ Candidates establish their "resting" heart rate and "working" heart rate. What is a good heart rate range for them? How might heart rate change for a baby? For a child? For an adult? What does heart rate tell candidates about the intensity of their workout?

❏ Encourage candidates to check their heart rate during fitness activities throughout their daily lives and adjust the activity accordingly.

▋ Blindfolds

Blindfold two volunteers. Choose some of the remaining candidates to perform a fitness activity that will increase their heart beat. The others remain inactive so their heart rate remains at resting level. Challenge blindfolded volunteers to determine who performed the fitness activity by monitoring pulse rate.

▋ Victim sim

Assign victim types. Include unconscious, injured, crying or distraught, and bleeding. Some candidates perform victim simulations, while others attempt to take their pulse. Switch roles.

Variations

❏ After the activity, discuss the experience. What did "rescuers" do that helped make it easier to take the person's pulse? Which victim types were most difficult?

(cont'd)

Notes

CPR: adult

▮ Manikins

Use manikins especially designed for CPR to practice proper airway seals, chest compressions and inflating victims' lungs. Emphasize why manikins are used for chest compression practice, and never "real people."

Variations

❏ Assist candidates to make their own CPR manikin. Assign homework to demonstrate CPR to a family member.

❏ Manikins designed for CPR practice (like ACTAR manikins) are recommended, but not mandatory. If these are not available, try a homemade manikin. For example, practice with a pillow and an old pillowcase. Draw the thorax on the pillowcase for landmarking and compressions.

▮ Step by step

Set up stations that feature the steps in the CPR sequence. Use one side of a long wall to give an overall view of the sequence. Post steps and related tasks at each station. Candidates visit the stations in order, beginning with assessment of hazards.

Variations

❏ Candidates work through the stations in pairs and practice the item (excluding chest compressions) on their partner. Place manikins at stations featuring chest compressions.

❏ Use a telephone and a tape recorder to practice accessing emergency medical services. Candidates listen to what they said to request help and evaluate effectiveness.

❏ At each station, candidates repeat the steps from the previous stations and add on the new step until they have "built" the entire skill and have had maximum practice.

▮ It's a rap

Challenge candidates to create a rap, a song, or a poem to help them remember the steps in CPR.

Variations

❏ Do the activity in pairs or small groups. Have candidates perform their rap, song, or poem for each other.

❏ Take the "show on the road!" Perform for others!

Learning Activities
Medical Emergencies

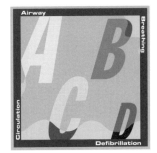

Variations

❏ Candidates bring a poison from home and relate to the group the signs & symptoms it could cause as well as the treatment.

❏ Instructor tries to stump the class with a common, everyday item (i.e. vitamins).

Jeopardy

In teams or individually, candidates choose the Medical Emergency category and must give the correct question to the answer.

Variations

❏ In teams, candidates prepare their own answers to challenge the other team.

Special guest

Invite an expert from the Epilepsy Foundation, Anaphylaxis Society or other related agency to do a presentation to the class.

Variations

❏ Ask someone who has a serious allergy or is a diabetic, to speak to the class.

To poison or not to poison

Prepare a table with a variety of empty containers (e.g., liquid bleach, detergent, shampoo, make-up, plant). Candidates write down all the poisons they can identify.

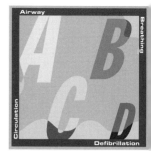

Learning Activities
Heat & Cold-related Emergencies

Classroom practice

Provide classroom practice of recognition and emergency care.

Treatment includes application of heat (personal body heat, etc.) or cold (ice) where appropriate, airway management and positioning of victims.

Simulations

Build a simulated severe burn progressing through 1st, 2nd and 3rd degree burns. Discuss prevention, causes and treatment.

Suggestions

❑ Refer to *Instructor Notes.*

❑ Provide a base of cold cream. Add red lipstick for 1st degree, Vaseline in globs covered with plastic wrap for 2nd and black Play-Doh™ for 3rd.

First Aid Test Answer Sheet

Emergency First Aid – *Answer Questions 1–25*   **Standard First Aid** – *Answer Questions 1–50*

Candidate name: _____

- Choose a single response for each question. The choice you make should correspond to the best way of answering the question, even if in certain cases there are partially correct choices.
- Mark your answer on this Answer Sheet. Do not write on the question paper.
- When finished, return the question paper together with the completed Answer Sheet.
- You may consult reference materials.
- Pass = minimum 70% (17/25 for Emergency First Aid or 35/50 for Standard First Aid).

EMERGENCY FIRST AID 1–25   ## STANDARD FIRST AID 1–50

1. a b c d	14. a b c d	26. a b c d	39. a b c d
2. a b c d	15. a b c d	27. a b c d	40. a b c d
3. a b c d	16. a b c d	28. a b c d	41. a b c d
4. a b c d	17. a b c d	29. a b c d	42. a b c d
5. a b c d	18. a b c d	30. a b c d	43. a b c d
6. a b c d	19. a b c d	31. a b c d	44. a b c d
7. a b c d	20. a b c d	32. a b c d	45. a b c d
8. a b c d	21. a b c d	33. a b c d	46. a b c d
9. a b c d	22. a b c d	34. a b c d	47. a b c d
10. a b c d	23. a b c d	35. a b c d	48. a b c d
11. a b c d	24. a b c d	36. a b c d	49. a b c d
12. a b c d	25. a b c d	37. a b c d	50. a b c d
13. a b c d		38. a b c d	

LIFESAVING SOCIETY

First Aid Test Answer Key

Emergency First Aid – *Answer Questions 1–25*   **Standard First Aid** – *Answer Questions 1–50*

- Choose a single response for each question. The choice you make should correspond to the best way of answering the question, even if in certain cases there are partially correct choices.

- Mark your answer on this Answer Sheet. Do not write on the question paper.

- When finished, return the question paper together with the completed Answer Sheet.

- You may consult reference materials.

- Pass = minimum 70% (17/25 for Emergency First Aid or 35/50 for Standard First Aid).

EMERGENCY FIRST AID 1–25

1. a b c **X**	14. a **X** c d
2. **X** b c d	15. a **X** c d
3. a **X** c d	16. a b c **X**
4. a b c **X**	17. a b c **X**
5. **X** b c d	18. a b c **X**
6. a b c **X**	19. a **X** c d
7. a b **X** d	20. a b c **X**
8. a b c **X**	21. **X** b c d
9. **X** b c d	22. **X** b c d
10. a b c **X**	23. a b **X** d
11. a b **X** d	24. a **X** c d
12. a **X** c d	25. **X** b c d
13. a **X** c d	

STANDARD FIRST AID 1–50

26. a **X** c d	39. a b c **X**
27. **X** b c d	40. a b c **X**
28. a **X** c d	41. a b **X** d
29. **X** b c d	42. a b c **X**
30. a b c **X**	43. a b c **X**
31. a b **X** d	44. a **X** c d
32. a **X** c d	45. a b c **X**
33. **X** b c d	46. **X** b c d
34. a b **X** d	47. **X** b c d
35. **X** b c d	48. a b c **X**
36. a **X** c d	49. a b c **X**
37. **X** b c d	50. a b c **X**
38. a **X** c d	

LIFESAVING SOCIETY

First Aid Test

Emergency First Aid – *Answer Questions 1–25*

1. You may start treatment on a victim when:
   a. The victim is unconscious
   b. The victim is a small child with no guardian present
   c. You ask for permission and the victim consents to treatment
   d. All of the above

2. You may stop treatment on a victim when:
   a. Medical help takes over
   b. The victim vomits
   c. The victim's heart stops beating
   d. All of the above

3. What do you do first when responding to an unwitnessed, unconscious child?
   a. Do a foreign body check
   b. Assess the environment for hazards
   c. Activate EMS
   d. Open the airway

4. What are the "3 Ps" of First Aid?
   a. Popular, principle and promote
   b. Produce, pronounce and prepare
   c. Principle, prevent and preserve
   d. Preserve, prevent and promote

5. In a primary assessment, if a drowning victim is unresponsive and non-breathing, you give 2 rescue breaths and start chest compressions.
   a. True
   b. False

Standard First Aid – *Answer Questions 1–50*

6. When you send a bystander to call EMS, the information he or she should provide is:
   a. The location of (and direction to) the incident
   b. The number of victims
   c. The victim's condition
   d. All of the above

7. Why is it important to use barrier devices (gloves, pocket mask) when doing CPR?
   a. To protect the victim
   b. To protect yourself
   c. To protect you and the victim
   d. To protect the environment

8. For which of the following would you use gloves?
   a. Nose bleed
   b. Heart attack
   c. Vomit
   d. All of the above

9. Somebody suffering from shock may look:
   a. Confused, pale and restless
   b. Excited, flushed and a strong regular pulse
   c. Scared, weak and hungry
   d. None of the above

10. What should you do for victims suffering from shock?
    a. Reassure them
    b. Call EMS
    c. Keep them warm and monitor their vitals
    d. All of the above

11. If a wound continues to bleed through a dressing bandage, you should:
    a. Remove the dressing and apply a clean one
    b. Lower the bleeding part further if possible
    c. Apply another dressing on top of the old one
    d. Do both a and b

12. If you are alone, when should you activate EMS for a 6-year-old unresponsive victim?
    a. Immediately
    b. After about 2 minutes of CPR
    c. After about 1 minute of CPR
    d. It is not necessary to activate EMS

13. If your conscious adult victim is choking and cannot speak or cough, you should first:
    a. Give 2 full breaths
    b. Give back blows/abdominal thrusts
    c. Do a finger sweep
    d. Activate EMS

14. If your choking victim goes unconscious, you should immediately:
    a. Assess the environment
    b. Activate EMS
    c. Reassess airway, breathing and circulation
    d. Reassure the victim

15. The appropriate ratio of chest compressions to breaths for an unconscious, choking adult is:
    a. 3:1
    b. 30:2
    c. 5:1
    d. 15:2

16. You should put an unconscious victim in recovery (semi-prone) position because:
    a. This is the best position in which to do mouth-to-mouth
    b. This is the best position in which to take a pulse
    c. This is the best position in which to check breathing
    d. This is the best position in which to allow vomit to drain

17. Which of the following are acceptable methods of doing rescue breathing?
    a. Mouth to mouth
    b. Mouth to nose
    c. Mouth to stoma
    d. All of the above

18. If a drowing victim's vomit blocks the airway, you should:
    a. Stop rescue breathing because the victim will start to breathe
    b. Continue rescue breathing
    c. Place the victim in recovery position and stop resuscitation
    d. Place the victim in recovery position and clear the airway

19. For a conscious, asthmatic victim with medication, you should:
    a. Force the administration of medication
    b. Assist the victim to take his medication
    c. Not allow administration of medication
    d. Not worry about medication until EMS arrives

20. What are some signs and symptoms of a heart attack?
    a. Chest pain and nausea
    b. Flushed face and sweating
    c. Chest pain, shortness of breath and denial
    d. All of the above

21. A stroke is similar to a heart attack, except that it involves the blood vessels which supply the brain:
    a. True
    b. False

22. Jo-Ann's grandmother is having weakness in her left arm and left leg. She is also anxious and disoriented. Jo-Ann should:
    a. Assist her into a comfortable position and call EMS
    b. Walk her to the bus stop
    c. Call EMS and start CPR
    d. Treat for shock

23. The ratio of compressions to breaths for one-rescuer adult CPR is:
    a. 5:1
    b. 15:2
    c. 30:2
    d. 1:1

24. You do not need to call EMS if an AED unit is on site with trained personnel.
    a. True
    b. False

25. A puncture or stab wound should be treated:
    a. As external bleeding
    b. Like CPR
    c. As a minor injury of low priority
    d. By EMS personnel only

EMERGENCY FIRST AID TEST
STOP HERE

26. A mother comes to you with a conscious choking infant. When should you send mom to activate EMS?
    a. After the infant goes unconscious
    b. While you are treating the infant
    c. After 2 minutes of CPR
    d. None of the above

27. The ratio of chest compressions to breaths for one-rescuer, infant CPR is 30:2.
    a. True
    b. False

28. If you are alone with no cell phone and find an unresponsive non-breathing infant, you should:
    a. Leave the infant and go call EMS as quickly as possible
    b. Perfom CPR (2 min.) and take infant with you to call EMS
    c. Reassess breathing every 20 seconds
    d. None of the above

29. A temporary chest pain that can be brought on by increased physical activity, stress or agitation is called:
    a. Angina
    b. Pedal edema
    c. Pulmonary edema
    d. Rhinoplasty

30. In two-person CPR, when the second rescuer arrives, she should:
    a. identify herself as knowing CPR
    b. check for bleeding
    c. confirm that EMS has been called
    d. a and c

31. A compound (or open) fracture is:
    a. A bone that is fractured in more than one location
    b. A bone that is broken in more than one location
    c. A bone that has broken through the skin
    d. A bone that has separated from the joint socket

32. Signs and symptoms of hypothermia are:
    a. Shivering; very active; shock
    b. Shivering; loss of muscle coordination; confusion
    c. Sweating profusely; red skin; unconsciousness
    d. Blood loss; nausea; dryness

33. When treating heat stroke, you need to remember to contact EMS and cool the victim down.
    a. True
    b. False

34. How many degrees of burns are there?
    a. One
    b. Two
    c. Three
    d. Four

35. A second degree burn is:
    a. Red, blistered and painful
    b. Black and charred
    c. Red, cool to the touch, itchy
    d. Treated best with butter

36. Loss of recent memory, disorientation, nausea and fluid from ears or nose are all signs of:
    a. Angina
    b. Head injury
    c. Broken bone
    d. Indigestion

37. A head injury that includes signs of bleeding, fluid discharge and skin damage should be treated with immobilization of the spine.
    a. True
    b. False

38. When treating a nosebleed, you should:
    a. Tilt the head back
    b. Pinch nose, tilt head forward
    c. Blow the nose
    d. Apply pressure to back of neck

39. A secondary assessment involves:
    a. Assessing and recording vital signs
    b. Carrying out a thorough head-to-toe examination of the victim
    c. Recording the relevant history
    d. All of the above

40. Chest wounds include injuries to the chest wall and ribs. These may include:
    a. Bruising
    b. Fractures
    c. Bleeding wounds
    d. All of the above

41. When treating an internal abdominal injury, you want to make sure you:
    a. Press hard on the injured area
    b. Give hot compress
    c. Contact EMS
    d. Make victim do sit-ups to exercise weak muscles

42. A hockey player falls head first into the boards. She can't feel her hands or her feet. As the rescuer you should:
    a. Remove the helmet, check the body
    b. Get bystanders to help move her off the ice to continue the game
    c. Call EMS, remove the helmet and perform CPR
    d. Call EMS, don't move her, monitor airway, breathing and circulation

43. Whether or not a spinal injury should be suspected can be based on:
    a. Mechanism of injury
    b. Questioning the victim or bystanders about what happened
    c. A head to toe examination that reveals signs and symptoms associated with spinal injuries
    d. All of the above

44. If a victim is having a seizure, you should place something between his teeth to prevent the victim from biting his tongue.
    a. True
    b. False.

45. Signs and symptoms of seizures may include:
    a. Loss of consciousness
    b. Arching of the back and rigidity of the body
    c. Loss of bladder control
    d. Any of the above

46. If you suspect a responsive victim is having a diabetic reaction, you should:
    a. give him pop or juice containing sugar
    b. ask him if he has a test kit
    c. administer insulin
    d. b and c

47. When dealing with a dental injury, a rescuer should try to salvage any lost or broken teeth.
    a. True
    b. False

48. You can be poisoned in the following way:
    a. Absorption
    b. Injection
    c. Ingestion
    d. All of the above

49. You can get first aid information regarding a certain ingested chemical by:
    a. Asking your mother
    b. Reading container information
    c. Contacting poison control centre
    d. b and c

50. After a rescue, support groups are available to address Critical Incidence Stress, for:
    a. All people involved in a successful rescue
    b. All people involved in an unsuccessful rescue
    c. There are no support groups, everyone can cope well with a rescue
    d. a and b

STANDARD FIRST AID TEST
STOP HERE